BIOCHEMICAL BASIS OF INHERITED HUMAN DISEASE

Papers by

Shintaro Okada, Harvey S. Singer, John S. O'Brien, David K. Kaplan, Gideon Bach, Mae Wan Ho, John C. Crawhall, Leo, Zelkowitz, Dominique Meyer, N. K. Day, C. J. Brackenridge, Terry Langer, Alfred G. Knudson, Jr., Stephen D. Litwin, G. F. Smith, L. Wetterberg, J. H. Renwick et al.

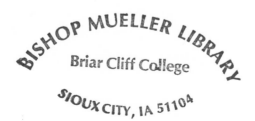
MSS Information Corporation
655 Madison Avenue, New York, N.Y. 10021

Library of Congress Cataloging in Publication Data
Main entry under title:

Biochemical basis of inherited human disease.

    CONTENTS: Okada, Veath, Leroy and O'Brien.
Ganglioside GM, storage disease: hexosaminidase
deficiencies in cultured fibroblasts.--Okada and
O'Brien. Tay-Sachs disease: generalized absence of
a beta-D-N-acetylhexosaminidase component. [etc.]
    1. Medical genetics--Addresses, essays, lectures.
I. Okada, Shintaro. [DNLM: 1. Genetics, Biochemical
--Collected works. 2. Hereditary diseases--Collected
works. QZ 50 B615 1973]
RB155.B49   616'.042'08   72-13557
ISBN 0-8422-7087-6

TABLE OF CONTENTS

CREDITS AND ACKNOWLEDGEMENTS

Bach, Gideon; Robert Friedman; Bernard Weissmann; and Elizabeth F. Neufeld, "The Defect in the Hurler and Scheie Syndromes: Deficiency of Alpha-L-Iduronidase," *Proceedings of the National Academy of Sciences*, 1972, 69:2048-2051.

Brackenridge, C.J., "A Genetic and Statistical Study of Some Sex-Related Factors in Huntington's Disease," *Clinical Genetics*, 1971, 2:267-286.

Brackenridge, C.J., "The Relation of Type of Initial Symptoms and Line of Transmission to Ages at Onset and Death in Huntington's Disease," *Clinical Genetics*, 1971, 2:287-297.

Crawhall, John C.; and Marianne Banfalvi, "Fabry's Disease: Differentiation Between Two Forms of an Alpha-Galactosidase by Myo-inositol," *Science*, 1972, 177:527-528.

Day, N.K.; H. Geiger; R. Stroud; M. deBracco; B. Mancado; D. Windhorst; and R.A. Good, "Clr Deficiency: An Inborn Error Associated with Cutaneous and Renal Disease," *The Journal of Clinical Investigation*, 1972, 51:1102-1108.

Ho, Mae Wan; Steven Beutler; Linda Tennant; and John S. O'Brien, "Fabry's Disease: Evidence for a Physically Altered Alpha-Galactosidase," *The American Journal of Human Genetics*, 1972, 24:256-266.

Kaplan, David, "Classification of the Mucopolysaccharidoses Based on the Pattern of Mucopolysacchariduria," *American Journal of Medicine*, 1969, 47:721-729.

Knudson, Jr., Alfred G., "Mutation and Cancer: Statistical Study of Retinoblastoma," *Proceedings of the National Academy of Sciences*, 1971, 68:820-823.

Langer, Terry; Warren Strober; and Robert I. Levy, "The Metabolism of Low Density Lipoprotein in Familial Type II Hyperlipoproteinemia," *The Journal of Clinical Investigation*, 1972, 51:1528-1536.

Litwin, Stephen D.; and H. Hugh Fudenberg, "Quantitative Abnormalities of Allotypic Genes in Families with Primary Immune Deficiencies," *Proceedings of the National Academy of Sciences*, 1972, 69:1739-1743.

Meyer, Dominique; Ethel Bidwell; and Marie José Larrieu, "Cross-Reacting Material in Genetic Variants of Haemophilia B," *Journal of Clinical Pathology*, 1972, 24:433-436.

O'Brien, John S., "Sanfilippo Syndrome: Profound Deficiency of Alpha-Acetylglucosaminidase Activity in Organs and Skin Fibroblasts from Type-B Patients," *Proceedings of the National Academy of Sciences,* 1972, 69:1720-1722.

Okada, Shintaro; M. Lois Veath; Jules Leroy; and John S. O'Brien, Ganglioside GM_2 Storage Diseases: Hexosaminidase Deficiencies in Cultured Fibroblasts," *The American Journal of Human Genetics,* 1971, 23:55-61.

Okada, Shintaro; and John S. O'Brien, "Tay-Sachs Disease: Generalized Absence of a Beta-D-N-Acetylhexosaminidase Component," *Science,* 1969, 165:698-700.

Renwick, J.H.; and D.R. Bolling, "An Analysis Procedure Illustrated on a Triple Linkage of Use for Prenatal Diagnosis of Myotonic Dystrophy," *Journal of Medical Genetics,* 1971, 8:399-406.

Renwick, J.H.; Sarah E. Bundey; M.A. Ferguson-Smith; and Marïan M. Izatt, "Confirmation of Linkage of the Loci for Myotonic Dystrophy and ABH Secretion," *Journal of Medical Genetics,* 1971, 8: 407-416.

Singer, Harvey S.; and Irwin A. Schafer, "Clinical and Enzymatic Variations in GM_1 Generalized Gangliosidosis," *The American Journal of Human Genetics,* 1972, 24:454-463.

Smith, G.F.; Parvin Justice; and D.Y.Y. Hsia, "Blood Enzymes in the de Lange Syndrome," *Journal of Medical Genetics,* 1972, 9:172-173.

Wetterberg, L.; K.-H. Gustavson; M. Bäckström; S.B. Ross; and Ö. Frödén, "Low Dopamine-B-Hydroxylase Activity in Down's Syndrome," *Clinical Genetics,* 1972, 3:152-153.

Zelkowitz, Leo; Claudio Torres; Nirmala Bhoopalam; Vincent J. Yakulis; and Paul Heller, "Double Heterozygous Beta-Sigma-Thalassemia in Negroes," *Archives of Internal Medicine,* 1972, 129:975-979.

PREFACE

Genetic disease is one of the few areas where biochemical geneticists have a direct impact on the treatment of patients. The most impressive achievements have come in the management of Phenylketonuria and galactosemia, where control of the disease and the abrogation of its severest effects have resulted from an understanding of the biochemical basis of the disorder.

Investigations of these diseases have taken two forms relating to patient care. These are prenatal detection, made possible by the development of amniocentesis and the improvements in culturing human tissue *in vitro* and an understanding of the metabolic pathways affected by the lesion, thereby enabling replacement or control of the defect. The first allows abortion of the fetus, preferably early in pregnancy, while the second leads to rational management of affected patients, either through dietary supervision or other environmental control.

This collection encompasses the most important recent findings in order to provide a basis for future investigations rather than merely cataloging the symptomology of inherited disorders, we have concentrated on the biochemical nature of the disease, in an attempt to pin point the genetic lesion and to separate it from the secondary effects that often accompany these syndromes. This has been the most fruitful approach in terms of both understanding the etiology of the symptoms, and constructing rational treatment schemes.

Jeffrey A. Frelinger, Ph.D.
Ronald T. Acton, Ph.D.
January, 1973

Ganglioside Disease

Ganglioside GM₂ Storage Diseases: Hexosaminidase Deficiencies in Cultured Fibroblasts

SHINTARO OKADA,[1] M. LOIS VEATH, JULES LEROY, AND JOHN S. O'BRIEN

INTRODUCTION

Ganglioside GM₂ is stored in three inborn errors of ganglioside metabolism, Tay-Sachs disease, Sandhoff's disease, and juvenile GM₂ gangliosidosis. Each appears to be transmitted as an autosomal recessive trait. Hexosaminidase A is absent in Tay-Sachs disease [1], both hexosaminidase A and B are absent in Sandhoff's disease [2], and a partial deficiency of hexosaminidase A has been demonstrated in juvenile GM₂ gangliosidosis [3, 4]. Descriptions of each disease are presented in a recent review [5]. We report here deficiencies of hexosaminidase components in cultured fibroblasts from patients with these three diseases, and document intermediate enzymic deficiencies in their parents.

MATERIALS AND METHODS

Skin biopsies were taken aseptically from the forearm or subscapular region after subcutaneous infiltration with 1% xylocaine. Specimens were immediately placed in sterile tubes containing medium F10, to which antibiotics and 15% fetal calf serum were added (Grand Island Biological Company). Biopsies were cut into 1–2-mm pieces, placed in 35-mm petri dishes under a cover slip, and 2 ml of the above medium was added. Petri dishes were then placed in an incubator maintained at 37° C, in an atmosphere of 95% oxygen and 5% carbon dioxide saturated with water vapor. Cultures were fed three times a week. After sufficient cell growth had occurred to cover the dish with a monolayer of outgrowing fibroblasts (two and one-half to three weeks), cells were subcultured by treatment with 0.25% trypsin. Frozen cell lines were obtained by freezing at the rate of 1° per minute in media containing 10% glycerol. Cells were stored in liquid nitrogen in glass ampules.

Enzyme assays were carried out on cell lines which had been subcultured at least once. Cells were harvested for assay by replacing the media with 0.85% saline, scraping the cells from the surface of the petri dish with a rubber policeman, centrifuging the cells at 3,000 RPM, and discarding the supernatant. Harvested cell lines could be stored frozen at −20° C prior to assay without affecting the activity of the enzymes studied here.

Portions of this study were supported by National Multiple Sclerosis grant no. 450, National Cystic Fibrosis Foundation grant, National Institutes of Health grant NB 08682, National Foundation for Neuromuscular Diseases grant-in-aid, Futures for Children-Los Angeles, Quick Children bequest, donation from the Children's Brain Diseases, National Institutes of Health Program project grant GM 17702-01, and a grant from the Belgian government to Jules Leroy.

The β-D-N-acetylglucosaminidase activity was assayed according to the procedure described previously by Okada and O'Brien [1]. The wet weight of the cultured skin fibroblasts was obtained and cells were frozen and thawed 20 times prior to homogenization in a ground glass Tenbroeck homogenizer in 10 volumes of distilled water. (One volume is equivalent to 1 g wet weight of cells per milliliter of homogenate.) Two microliter aliquots of the fibroblast homogenate were taken and diluted with 20 μliter of 0.04 M citrate phosphate buffer (pH 4.3). To each sample was added 60 nanomoles of 4-methylumbelliferyl-β-D-N-acetylglucosamine (Pierce Co.) dissolved in 20 μliter of the same citrate-phosphate buffer described above. Samples were then incubated at 37° C for 15 and 30 minutes. The reaction

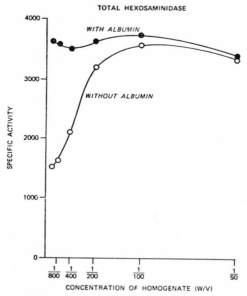

TOTAL HEXOSAMINIDASE

FIG. 1.—Effect of dilution of fibroblast homogenate with buffer on hexosaminidase-specific activity (nanomoles of 4-methylumbelliferyl-β-D-N-acetylglucosamine cleaved per milligram protein per hour). Lower curve—specific activity at varying concentrations of homogenate in buffer in the absence of albumin. Upper curve—0.1% human serum albumin added to each sample prior to assay.

was terminated by adding 2.5 ml of 0.17 M glycine-carbonate buffer (pH 10). Fluorescence was read in a Turner fluorometer at an excitation wavelength of 365 mμ and an emission wavelength of 450 mμ. Protein determinations were carried out by the method of Lowry et al. [6].

It was found that if dilute fibroblast homogenates (greater than one in 200) were used for enzyme assay, the hexosaminidase activity was lower than in concentrated homogenates (fig. 1). Addition of human serum albumin (grade III, Sigma Co.) to dilute homogenates resulted in the restoration of activity to levels found in concentrated homogenates (fig. 1). For this reason, 0.075% human serum albumin was routinely added to all homogenates. Optimal enzyme activity occurred at a concentration of 0.05%–0.1% albumin. At concentrations less than 0.05%, activity rapidly fell. The human albumin used had negligible hexosaminidase activity.

11

Hexosaminidase A and hexosaminidase B were quantified by a method which exploits the different thermal stabilities of each [7]. This method, devised for human serum, was used essentially unchanged for fibroblasts except for the addition of 0.075% serum albumin to each homogenate.

Starch gel electrophoresis studies were carried out on aliquots of skin fibroblast homogenates according to the method of Okada and O'Brien [1]. Hexosaminidase A and hexosaminidase B were detected by the fluorescence produced after incubation of the gels with 4-methylumbelliferyl-β-D-N-acetylglucosamine. The results of the electrophoretic experiments confirmed the quantitative studies (fig. 2). Both hexosaminidase A and B were present in cultured fibroblasts from controls, and approximately half the activity was due to hexosaminidase A. Hexosaminidase A was absent in cultured fibroblasts from patients with Tay-Sachs disease. Both hexosaminidase A and B were undetected in the fibroblasts from the patient with Sandhoff's disease. Fibroblasts from a patient with juvenile GM_2 gangliosidosis had a reduced, but not totally absent, activity of hexosaminidase A.

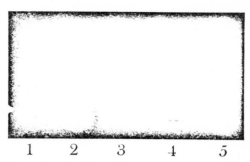

FIG. 2.—Starch gel electrophoresis of hexosaminidases from skin fibroblasts of patients with ganglioside GM_2 storage diseases. Upper spot is hexosaminidase A, lower spot, hexosaminidase B. Twenty μliter of a one-in-10 homogenate was applied to each slot. Control subjects—slots 1 and 5, Tay-Sachs disease patient—slot 2, Sandhoff's disease patient—slot 3, and juvenile GM_2 gangliosidosis patient—slot 4. Hexosaminidase A was clearly visible on the original gel in sample 4, but did not photograph well.

Subjects studied in this report included 20 control subjects, ranging in age from birth to 46 years. Also studied were eight parents of children with Tay-Sachs disease, five children with Tay-Sachs disease, one child with Sandhoff's disease and his mother, and five members of a family (mother, father, patient, brother, and sister) in which the oldest girl had juvenile GM_2 gangliosidosis.

RESULTS

The specific activity of total hexosaminidase (A plus B) varied according to the growth of the culture (fig. 3). Immediately after subculture, a drop in hexosaminidase activity occurred, with the lowest activity four days after subculture. Specific activity increased progressively to 22 days and then leveled off. The cultures were heavily confluent by examination at 10 days after subculture. The total protein content per culture dish (fig. 4) increased linearly over the same time period.

The ratio of hexosaminidase A to hexosaminidase B did not change appreciably during the growth of the culture (fig. 5). The activity of hexosaminidase A in skin fibroblasts from the parent of a child with Tay-Sachs disease averaged approximately 60% of normal at all stages of growth (fig. 5).

To minimize variation of enzyme activity resulting from culture growth, all cultures were harvested for enzyme assay at 21–30 days after subculture. Total hexosaminidase activity in the fibroblasts from patients with Tay-Sachs disease, their parents, a patient with juvenile GM_2 gangliosidosis, and her parents fell within the range of controls (fig. 6). Total hexosaminidase activity in the patient

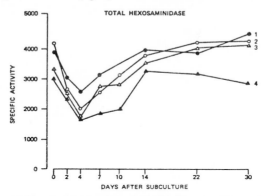

Fig. 3.—Hexosaminidase activity in cultured skin fibroblasts at different days after subculture. Strain 1—normal four-year-old girl, strain 2—parent of child with Tay-Sachs disease, strain 3—40-year-old woman with mental retardation, and strain 4—foreskin from normal newborn boy. Specific activity is expressed as nanomoles cleaved per milligram protein per hour.

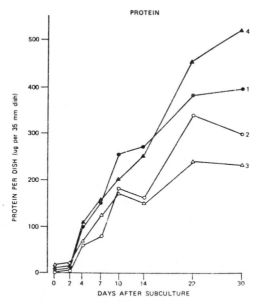

Fig. 4.—Protein content per culture dish at different days after subculture. For identification of strains, see figure 3.

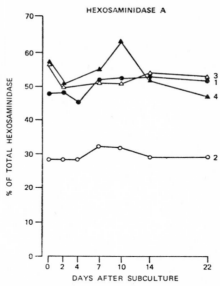

FIG. 5.—Hexosaminidase A activity at different days after subculture expressed as percentage of the total hexosaminidase. For identification of strains, see figure 3.

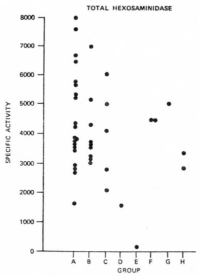

FIG. 6.—Total hexosaminidase activity in skin fibroblasts three weeks or more after subculture. Group A—controls, B—parents of patients with Tay-Sachs disease, C—patients with Tay-Sachs disease, D—mother of patient with Sandhoff's disease, E—patient with Sandhoff's disease, F—parents of patient with juvenile GM₂ gangliosidosis, G—patient with juvenile GM₂ gangliosidosis, and H—siblings of patient with juvenile GM₂ gangliosidosis.

14

with Sandhoff's disease was less than 5% of the control values. Activities in this patient's mother averaged 35% of the mean of control values.

In control subjects, hexosaminidase A comprised 49% ± 6% of the total hexosaminidase (fig. 7). In eight parents of children with Tay-Sachs disease, hexosaminidase A comprised 23% of the total hexosaminidase. In five children with Tay-Sachs disease, the value was 3.4% of the total hexosaminidase. There was no overlap between the values obtained from control subjects, heterozygotes, and homozygotes. The nearly normal activity of total hexosaminidase in cells from children with Tay-Sachs disease is due to a two-fold elevation of hexosaminidase B. In the cells

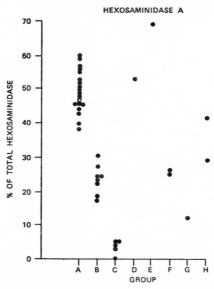

Fig. 7.—Hexosaminidase A activity in skin fibroblasts three weeks or more after subculture. For identification of groups, see figure 6.

from the boy with Sandhoff's disease and his mother, hexosaminidase A was deficient to the same extent as hexosaminidase B, thus the ratio of one to the other was nearly normal.

In the patient with juvenile GM₂ gangliosidosis, hexosaminidase A comprised 12% of the total hexosaminidase, a value 25% of normal. Both parents of the patient with juvenile GM₂ gangliosidosis had deficient levels of hexosaminidase A. Their values fell within the range of heterozygotes for Tay-Sachs disease. Two siblings of the patient were also assayed. One had deficient levels of hexosaminidase, indicating he is heterozygous; the other had normal levels.

DISCUSSION

Stage of culture influences the specific activity of hexosaminidase. A similar effect has been previously published by Leroy and DeMars [8] for another lysosomal

15

enzyme, β-glucuronidase. The increase in activity as the culture matures may reflect a change in metabolism from one in which cell division predominates to one in which more highly differentiated functions, including lysosomal hydrolase enzyme synthesis, become more important. This effect is important in establishing values for the specific activity of lysosomal enzymes in cell culture. It is especially important where enzyme-specific activity is used in diagnostic studies, such as amniocentesis and prenatal diagnosis. Control values must be established for cells which are at the same stage of culture as the patient's sample. As demonstrated here, the ratio of two closely related enzymes can be used to assess the deficiency of one or the other, as long as it is established that the relationship of the two is constant during different stages of culture growth.

These studies demonstrate the persistence of hexosaminidase deficiencies in cells derived from patients with each of the ganglioside GM_2 storage diseases. The fact that fibroblasts from parents of patients with each disease have intermediate reductions of enzyme activity is a further indication that the enzyme deficiency is a manifestation of the fundamental genetic defect in each. Diagnosis of homozygotes and detection of heterozygotes may be carried out on cultured cells. Fibroblast cultures will be useful in determining the relationship of the genetic defect to the enzymic abnormality in these inborn errors of ganglioside metabolism.

SUMMARY

Hexosaminidase A and hexosaminidase B were assayed in cultured skin fibroblasts derived from patients with three ganglioside GM_2 storage diseases (Tay-Sachs disease, Sandhoff's disease, and juvenile GM_2 gangliosidosis) and compared to controls. Stage of culture and conditions of enzyme assay markedly influenced enzyme activity. Both hexosaminidase A and B were diminished to less than 5% of control values in cells from a patient with Sandhoff's disease; cells from his mother had an intermediate deficiency of these enzymes. Hexosaminidase A was diminished to less than 10% of control values in cells from patients with Tay-Sachs disease; cells from their parents had intermediate deficiencies of this enzyme. Hexosaminidase A was diminished to 25% of control values in cells from a patient with juvenile GM_2 gangliosidosis; cells from her parents had intermediate deficiencies of this enzyme.

REFERENCES

1. OKADA S, O'BRIEN JS: Tay-Sachs disease: generalized absence of a β-D-N-acetylhexosaminidase component. *Science* 165:698–700, 1969
2. SANDHOFF K: Variation of β-N-acetylhexosaminidase pattern in Tay-Sachs disease. *Fed Europ Biochem Soc Letters* 4:351–354, 1969
3. O'BRIEN JS: Five gangliosidoses. *Lancet* 2:805, 1969
4. OKADA S, VEATH ML, O'BRIEN JS: Juvenile GM_2 gangliosidosis: partial deficiency of hexosaminidase A. *J Pediat.* In press, 1970
5. O'BRIEN JS: Ganglioside storage diseases. *Fed Proc.* In press, 1970
6. LOWRY O, ROSEBROUGH NJ, FARR AL, et al: Protein measurement with the folin phenol reagent. *J Biol Chem* 193:265–275, 1951
7. O'BRIEN JS, OKADA S, CHEN A, et al: Tay-Sachs disease: detection of homozygotes and heterozygotes by serum hexosaminidase assay. *New Eng J Med* 283:15–20, 1970
8. LEROY JG, DEMARS RI: Mutant enzymatic and cytological phenotypes in cultured human fibroblasts. *Science* 157:804–806, 1967

Tay-Sachs Disease: Generalized Absence of a Beta-D-N-Acetylhexosaminidase Component

SHINTARO OKADA
JOHN S. O'BRIEN

Tay-Sachs disease is a hereditary disorder transmitted as an autosomal recessive trait involving the massive cerebral accumulation of a specific ganglioside, GM_2 (*1*). The disease is invariably fatal; progressive cerebral degeneration results in death by the second, third, or fourth year of life (*2*). The ganglioside has a carbohydrate and a fatty acid composition identical to that of the normal cerebral ganglioside GM_2 (*1, 3*), namely, N-acetylgalactosaminyl-$(1 \rightarrow 4)$-[$(2 \rightarrow 3)$-N-acetylneuraminyl]-galactosyl-$(1 \rightarrow 4)$-glucosyl-$(1 \rightarrow 1)$-[2-N-acyl]-sphingosine.

The enzyme defect in Tay-Sachs disease is unknown. A degradative enzymic failure is a likely possibility (*4*). In generalized gangliosidosis, another ganglioside storage disease in which ganglioside GM_1 accumulates (*5*), Okada and O'Brien (*6*) have demonstrated a profound deficiency of a β-galactosidase which cleaves the terminal galactose from the stored ganglioside. Absence of a lysosomally localized hexosaminidase which cleaves the terminal N-acetylgalactosamine from the oligosaccharide moiety of ganglioside GM_2 could account for the degree and the localization of ganglioside accumulation in Tay-Sachs disease on a similar basis. Despite the satisfying nature of this explanation, hexosaminidase activities in cerebral tissues of patients with Tay-Sachs disease are elevated rather than deficient (*7*, Table 1) when assays are performed with synthetic substrates.

It seemed worth while to explore the physical properties and the electrophoretic behavior of hexosaminidases in Tay-Sachs disease in order to determine whether abnormalities of this enzyme might be present. This report documents the absence of a β-D-N-acetylhexosaminidase component in frozen organs, in blood plasma, and in living cells from patients with Tay-Sachs disease.

Tissues were available from seven patients (2 to 6 years of age, four boys, three girls) who died from Tay-Sachs disease. All tissues were stored at $-20°C$ prior to analysis; the activities of all enzymes studied here were not affected by prolonged (1 to 5 years)

17

Table 1. Acid hydrolase activity in Tay-Sachs disease (TSD). Values in brain, liver, and kidney are expressed as nanomoles of substrate cleaved per milligram of wet tissue per hour. Values in skin are expressed as nanomoles of substrate cleaved per milligram of protein per hour. Enzyme values in parentheses are the average values for each group.

Subjects	No.	β-Glucosidase	β-Galactosidase	β-N-Acetyl-glucos-aminidase	β-N-Acetyl-galactos-aminidase
			Cerebral cortex		
Controls	9	0.42–1.32 (0.82)	1.87–2.56 (2.19)	30.7–78.6 (50.5)	7.4–18.4 (12.9)
TSD	4	0.71–1.66 (1.30)	4.6–8.3 (5.8)	126.5–246.9 (157.9)	86.0–118.2 (98.6)
			Liver		
Controls	17	1.3–13.7 (5.8)	16.3–46.0 (30.3)	121–563 (323)	19.9–54.1 (41.0)
TSD	3	7.8–14.1 (10.9)	41.1–47.6 (44.2)	77–157 (106)	10.4–19.7 (14.4)
			Kidney		
Controls	2	4.0–7.6 (5.8)	42.0–47.2 (44.6)	273–344 (309)	35.3–54.9 (45.1)
TSD	3	9.5–12.2 (11.0)	66.7–76.2 (71.6)	136–287 (190)	14.5–36.0 (23.4)
			Skin		
Controls	22			52.8–285.6 (159)	16.4*
TSD	3			63.6–148.6 (105.8)	9.2–15.4 (12.8)

* A single assay only.

frozen storage of control tissues. Control tissues were obtained from 14 patients who died of disorders not involving the central nervous system, from two patients with late infantile amaurotic idiocy (Jansky-Bielschowsky type), from six patients with the Hurler's syndrome (mucopolysaccharidosis types 1 to 3), and from two patients with generalized gangliosidosis. Many of the controls were similar in age to the Tay-Sachs patients, and all tissues were stored for similar periods (1 to 5 years). Control patients with generalized gangliosidosis and late infantile amaurotic idiocy had taken anticonvulsants and antibiotics during the course of their illness, as had the Tay-Sachs patients.

Venous blood was obtained from two living patients, a 14-month-old boy and a 4-year-old girl, with Tay-Sachs disease and from five healthy adult subjects; leukocytes were isolated from 5 ml of whole blood after the erythrocytes were precipitated with dextran (8).

β-D-N-Acetylglucosaminidase and β-D-N-acetylgalactosaminidase activities were assayed at pH 4.4 in citrate-phosphate buffer (0.1M) with both p-nitrophenyl and 4-methylumbelliferyl derivatives (Pierce Co.) of the corresponding β-D-N-acetylhexosaminides as substrates (9). β-Galactosidase and β-glucosidase activities were assayed at pH 5.0 in acetate buffer (0.1M) with both the *p*-nitrophenyl and the 4-methylumbelliferyl derivates of each β-D-hexopyranoside (Pierce Co.) as substrates (*6, 10*). Assays were performed on tissue homogenates in distilled water and on supernatant fractions obtained by high speed centrifugation (100,000*g* for 60 minutes) of homogenates. Vertical starch-gel electrophoresis was performed by the method of Smithies (*11*) with the use of commercially available starch and apparatus (Otto Hiller, Madison, Wisconsin). The electrode buffer was varied between *p̄*H 5.0 and 7.6 (citrate-phosphate buffer 0.04*M*). After development, the gels were incubated with 4-methylumbelliferyl-β-D- derivatives of each substrate, and fluorescent regions of enzyme activity were located by viewing the gels under ultraviolet light after they were sprayed with alkali (glycine-carbonate buffer 0.25*M*, *p*H 9.8) to enhance fluorescence. Violet areas of hexosaminidase activity were obtained by incubating the gels at 37°C with the naphthol AS-BI derivatives of β-D-*N*-acetylglucosaminide (incubation time, 1 hour) and β-D-*N*-acetylgalactosaminide (incubation time, 4 hours) at *p*H 4.4 in 0.1*M* citrate-phosphate buffer according to Hayashi (*12*); violet spots appeared when the released naphthol AS-BI was coupled with Fast Garnet GBC salt (*o*-aminoazotoluene, diazonium salt, Sigma Co.) (1 mg/ml) in the same buffer, but at *p*H 7.5, for 1 hour. Quantification of each colored spot was made by densitometric analysis of the gels, with commercially available equipment (Photovolt densitometer). We used the densitometric method to quantify the relative proportions of individual hexosaminidase components in tissues and body fluids.

The activities of β-D-*N*-acetylglucos-aminidase, β-D-*N*-acetylgalactosaminidase, β-glucosidase, and β-galactosidase were elevated in the cerebral cortex of Tay-Sachs patients compared to controls (Table 1). The average activities of the β-D-*N*-acetylglucosaminidase and β-D-*N*-acetylgalactosaminidase in liver, kidney, and skin were lower in the Tay-Sachs patients compared to controls, but there was overlap between the two groups. The *p*H optimum of β-D-*N*-acetylglucosaminidase in liver tissue from controls and Tay-Sachs patients was identical (*p*H 4.4 in both groups).

The sedimentation properties of β-D-*N*-acetylglucosaminidase and β-D-*N*-acetylgalactosaminidase in Tay-Sachs tissues differed markedly from the controls. After high speed centrifugation (100,000*g* for 60 minutes) of brain homogenates, which had been frozen and thawed many times and diluted 1 to 20 with distilled water, a large proportion (85 percent) of the hexosaminidase activity from controls remained in the supernatant fraction. After the same treatment only 20 percent of the hexosaminidase activity in the brain homogenate from Tay-Sachs patients was present in the supernatant; 80 percent of the activity was in the sediment. Similar results were obtained with kidney tissue. The reason for this behavior became obvious after starch-gel electrophoresis of hexosaminidases. Starch-gel electrophoresis studies demonstrated that two major hexosaminidase components were present in all organs from control subjects (Fig. 1); one hexosaminidase (component A) migrated rapidly toward the node, and the other hexosaminidase (component B) migrated slowly toward the cathode at *p*H 6.0. Incubation of supernatant fractions or tissue homogenates overnight in 2*M* urea or 1*M* sodium chloride at 4°C did not result

Table 2. Activity of hexosaminidase components in Tay-Sachs disease. Values are expressed as nanomoles of substrate cleaved per milligram of wet tissue per hour. Values in parentheses are the percentages of the total hexosaminidase activity of each component.

Subjects	No.	β-N-Acetylglucosaminidase Component		β-N-Acetylgalactosaminidase Component	
		A	B	A	B
Cerebral cortex					
Controls	9	38.9 (77)	11.6 (23)	9.9	3.0
Tay-Sachs	4	0	157.9 (100)	0	98.6
Liver					
Controls	17	129.2 (40)	193.8 (60)	16.4	24.6
Tay-Sachs	3	0	106 (100)	0	14.4
Kidney					
Controls	2	123.6 (40)	185.4 (60)	18.0	27.1
Tay-Sachs	3	0	190 (100)	0	23.4

in an alteration of the relative proportions of the two components. Both components possessed β-D-N-acetylglucosaminidase and β-D-N-acetylgalactosaminidase activity, as demonstrated by incubating starch gels with the 4-methylumbelliferyl, p-nitrophenyl, and naphthol AS-BI derivatives of each β-D-N-acetylhexosaminide. However, the activity of β-D-N-acetylgalactosaminidase was approximately one-eighth that of β-D-N-acetylglucosaminidase. After high speed centrifugation of brain or kidney homogenates from control subjects as described above, component B occurred predominately in the sediment while component A occurred predominantly in the supernatant solution. Robinson and Stirling (13) have reported similar results from a study of hexosaminidase in human spleen and have demonstrated that the two hexosaminidase components possess similar K_m (Michaelis constant) values, are readily separated by chromatography on diethylaminoethyl-cellulose, and are both present in the lysosomal fraction. They also found that specificity for orientation on the 4-carbon was not absolute; both components isolated from human spleen possessed β-D-N-acetylglucosaminidase and β-D-N-acetylgalactosaminidase activity. Our results with human liver, brain, skin, and kidney agree with theirs.

Starch-gel electrophoresis studies of the hexosaminidases in Tay-Sachs disease demonstrated that component A was absent in all frozen tissues available (brain, liver, kidney, and skin). The absence of component A in the Tay-Sachs patients' tissues was demonstrated with both the p-nitrophenyl and the naphthol AS-BI derivatives of both β-D-N-acetylglucosamine and β-D-N-

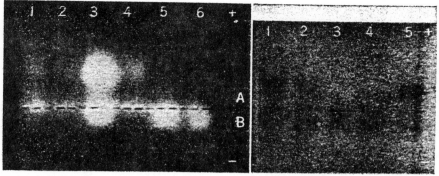

Fig. 1. Separation of β-D-N-acetylhexosaminidase components by starch-gel electrophoresis. The A components appear above the origin; the B components appear below the origin. (Left) Pattern in cerebral cortex (4-methylumbelliferyl-β-D-N-acetylglucosaminide as substrate) from patients with (1) late infantile amaurotic idiocy (aged 5); (2) renal disease (aged 6); (3) generalized gangliosidosis (aged 2); (4) carcinoma of lung (aged 59); (5) Tay-Sachs disease (aged 3); and (6) Tay-Sachs disease (aged 5). (Right) Pattern in leukocytes (naphthol-AS-BI-β-D-N-acetylglucosaminide as substrate) from (1) normal subject (aged 23); (2) normal subject (aged 22); (3) Tay-Sachs patient (aged 4); (4) Tay-Sachs patient (aged 14 months); and (5) normal subject (aged 23). Fifty microliters of a 1 to 20 homogenate was applied to each slot.

acetylgalactosamine as substrates, as well as 4-methylumbelliferyl-β-D-N-acetylglucosaminide. The activity of hexosaminidase component B was markedly increased in cerebral cortex from the Tay-Sachs patients compared to controls (Table 2), explaining the high levels of hexosaminidase activity in this tissue (Table 1), but hexosaminidase A was not detected.

In three other neuronal lipid storage disorders, generalized gangliosidosis, Hurler's syndrome, and late infantile amaurotic idiocy, no deficiency of hexosaminidase component A was found (Fig. 1). These results indicated that ganglioside storage in itself, neuronal lipidosis, slowly progressive fatal cerebral degeneration, and prolonged storage of frozen tissues were not responsible for the deficiency of hexosaminidase component A in the brain of Tay-Sachs patients.

It seemed unlikely that storage of ganglioside GM$_2$ in itself accounted for the deficiency of hexosaminidase A, since the deficiency was the same in brain, where ganglioside storage is massive, and in liver, kidney, and skin, where ganglioside storage is minimal.

When brain or liver homogenates from controls and Tay-Sachs patients were mixed in equal proportions, the activity of hexosaminidase component A in the mixed sample was the average of the control and Tay-Sachs activities. This finding indicated that soluble endogenous inhibitors (including ganglioside GM$_2$ which was soluble in the buffers used) were not responsible for the complete inactivity of component A.

21

Starch-gel electrophoretic studies of other glycohydrolases from cerebral gray matter and liver tissues of the Tay-Sachs patients revealed no alteration of enzyme patterns. This was true of β-galactosidase, which can be separated into three or four components in gray matter and in liver (*14*), as well as β-glucuronidase and β-glucosidase, which can be separated into two or three components (*15*).

Studies on fresh venous blood demonstrated that component A was the major hexosaminidase in normal human plasma and only traces of component B were present. Component A was absent in fresh plasma obtained from two living patients with Tay-Sachs disease; all the hexosaminidase activity was due to component B.

Leukocytes from control subjects contained both hexosaminidase components in the ratio of 73 percent A to 27 percent B. Leukocytes obtained fresh and assayed immediately from both living patients with Tay-Sachs disease contained component B; component A was absent (Fig. 1). Hexosaminidase A was absent in cultured skin fibroblasts (greater than ten cellular generations) obtained from three patients with Tay-Sachs disease; skin fibroblasts cultured from control subjects contained high concentrations of hexosaminidase A. Tay-Sachs fibroblasts contained normal concentrations of hexosaminidase B.

The absence of a β-D-N-acetylhexosaminidase component which possesses both N-acetyl-β-D-glucosaminidase and N-acetyl-β-D-galactosaminidase activity could provide a satisfactory explanation for the ganglioside storage in Tay-Sachs disease. A block in the catabolism of ganglioside GM_2, which contains a terminal N-acetylgalactosamine residue, could result from the absence of such a hydrolytic lysosomally localized enzyme. Before acceptance of this explanation, it must be demonstrated that hexosaminidase component A participates in the catabolism of ganglioside GM_2. Nonetheless, the fact that the deficiency occurs in all Tay-Sachs tissues studied and that levels of hexosaminidase A in plasma and leukocytes in heterozygous carriers of the Tay-Sachs gene are intermediate between homozygous affected patients and controls (*15*) suggests that the enzyme deficiency is closely related to the genetic defect.

The immediate practical importance of our discovery is that hexosaminidase assay provides a means for the diagnosis of homozygotes. We have found (*15*) that both hexosaminidase components are present in normal fetal amniotic fluid cells obtained by amniocentesis early in pregnancy. If component A is absent in fetal amniotic cells derived from individuals homozygous for Tay-Sachs disease, as appears likely, the intrauterine diagnosis of this fatal human disease will be possible.

References and Notes

1. L. Svennerholm, *Biochem. Biophys. Res. Commun.* 9, 436 (1962).
2. B. W. Volk, Ed., *Tay-Sachs Disease* (Grune and Stratton, New York, 1964).
3. R. Ledeen and K. Salsman, *Biochemistry* 4, 225 (1965).
4. R. O. Brady, *New Engl. J. Med.* 275, 312 (1966); L. Svennerholm, *Biochem. J.* 111, 6P (1969); H. Jatzkewitz and K. Sandhoff, *Biochim. Biophys. Acta* 70, 354 (1963).
5. J. S. O'Brien, M. B. Stern, B. H. Landing, J. K. O'Brien, G. N. Donnell, *Amer. J. Dis. Child.* 109, 338 (1965); N. K. Gonatas and J. Gonatas, *J. Neuropathol. Exp. Neurol.* 24, 318 (1965).
6. S. Okada and J. S. O'Brien, *Science* 160, 1002 (1968).

7. K. Sandhoff, U. Andreae, H. Jatzkewitz, *Life Sci.* **7**, 283 (1968).
8. P. J. Kampine, R. O. Brady, J. N. Kanfer, M. Feld, D. Shapiro, *Science* **155**, 86 (1966).
9. D. H. Leaback and P. G. Walker, *Biochem J.* **78**, 151 (1961); P. G. Walker, J. W. Woollen, R. Heyworth, *ibid.* **79**, 288. (1961).
10. S. Gatt and M. M. Rapport, *Biochim. Biophys. Acta* **113**, 567 (1966).
11. O. Smithies, *Biochem. J.* **71**, 585 (1958).
12. M. Hayashi, *J. Histochem. Cytochem.* **13**, 355 (1965).
13. D. Robinson and J. L. Stirling, *Biochem. J.* **107**, 321 (1965).
14. M. W. Ho and J. S. O'Brien, *Science* **165**, 611 (1969).
15. S. Okada, M. W. Ho, J. S. O'Brien, unpublished data.
16. We are indebted to Drs. C. Jacobson and J. E. Seegmiller for these cells. We thank Dr. H. Kihara and the staff of Pacific State Hospital, Pomona, California, for making the Tay-Sachs patients available and for supplying cultured skin fibroblasts. This work was supported by grants NB 06576 and HE 08428 from the National Institutes of Health.

Clinical and Enzymatic Variations in G_{M1} Generalized Gangliosidosis

HARVEY S. SINGER AND IRWIN A. SCHAFER

INTRODUCTION

Generalized gangliosidosis is a recessively inherited metabolic disorder characterized chemically by the storage of G_{M1} ganglioside in the brain and viscera plus the accumulation of a keratan sulfate–like polysaccharide in visceral tissues [1]. Two forms of the disease have been recognized clinically, based upon time of onset of symptoms and the degree of visceral storage and bone involvement. The early-onset (type 1) patient becomes ill early in infancy and resembles the infant with Hurler's syndrome with psychomotor retardation, hepatosplenomegaly, coarsening of facial features, and bone dysplasia. Children with the late-onset (type 2) form of the disease develop symptoms of progressive neurological deterioration beginning at 7–14 months but show only minimal evidence of visceral storage or bone disease [2]. These rather distinct clinical phenotypes coupled with the failure to observe both phenotypes in a single sibship suggest that the two clinical forms of G_{M1} gangliosidosis represent separate and distinct genetic diseases.

Chemically, the concentrations of cerebral G_{M1} ganglioside are similar in both type 1 and type 2 patients [3]. In other organs, type 2 patients generally store less G_{M1} ganglioside and polysaccharide than type 1 patients, but the correlation is not perfect [4]. The enzymatic basis for lysosomal storage in this disease has been related to a deficiency in the activity of one or more forms of the enzyme β-D-galactosidase, which normally cleaves the terminal galactose from the G_{M1} ganglioside [5]. This enzyme has also been implicated in the degradation of the keratan sulfate–like polysaccharide stored in liver [6].

If the degree of visceral storage in the two forms of the disease were related to mutations at different genetic loci, one would expect to find differences in the properties of β-galactosidase from type 1 and type 2 patients. The purpose of this study was to test this possibility in liver obtained by biopsy from two children with phenotypically distinct forms of G_{M1} gangliosidosis. We found that liver β-galactosidase in both the type 1 and type 2 patients had similar pH optima and identical patterns of activity on starch-gel electrophoresis suggesting a mutation at the same locus in both patients.

This work was supported by U.S. Public Health Service grant HD-03448 and a grant from the Cleveland Foundation.

24

Variations in the degree of visceral storage in individual patients may be related to the total activity of a pH 6.5 β-galactosidase which was markedly elevated in the type 2 patient.

METHODS

Preparation of Tissues

Hepatic β-galactosidase activity was assayed immediately after liver tissue was obtained. A 100–150 mg sample of tissue was homogenized in an ice bath using a Dounce glass hand grinder in 0.25 M sucrose containing 2.5% detergent (Cutscum Detergent, Fisher Scientific Company, Pittsburgh). The cellular homogenate was then centrifuged at 34,000 g for 20 min at 4° C, and the supernatant used for the enzyme assay.

Standard Enzyme Assay

Activity of β-galactosidase was assayed using p-nitrophenyl-β-D-galactopyranoside as substrate following a modification of the method described by Gatt and Rapport [7]. The reaction mixture consisted of 100 μl of 0.1 M acetate buffer (or 0.2 M lactate buffer adjusted to the desired pH), 2 μmoles of p-nitrophenyl-β-D-galactopyranoside in 100 μl of water, and 20 μl of hepatic enzyme supernate containing 50–100 μg of protein. Following incubation for 90 min at 37° C, the reaction was stopped with 100 μl of 1.0 M trichloroacetic acid. Then 2 ml cold absolute ethanol was added with shaking, and the tubes were centrifuged at 1,500 rpm for 10 min.

The clear alcohol supernatant was decanted and alkalinized with 1.5 ml of 0.2 M glycine-carbonate buffer, pH 10.7. The intense yellow color of free p-nitrophenol in alkaline solution was measured in a Bausch and Lomb Spectronic 20 at 410 mμ. Appropriate controls were used with each assay to rule out nonspecific hydrolysis and to correct for interfering color.

Enzyme activity was expressed as nanomoles of p-nitrophenyl-β-D-galactopyranoside hydrolyzed per hour per milligram of wet weight of tissue. Because differences in the degree of hepatic storage could introduce artifact in data expressed on a wet-weight basis, enzyme activities were checked using soluble supernatant protein as the denominator. Protein was measured by a modification of the method of Lowry et al. [8], in which the $CuSO_4$ was stabilized in alkaline solution with disodium EDTA (W. Robertson and B. Van, personal communication).

Conditions for the Standard Assay

The conditions for the assay of β-galactosidase activity in liver homogenates and partially purified enzyme preparations have been studied by several investigators [9–11] and were again confirmed in our laboratory.

The rate of hydrolysis of substrate at pH 3.6 and 6.5 was linear through 120 min incubation at 37° C using 25, 50, 75, 100, and 150 μg of protein in the supernatant prepared from normal tissue homogenates. A 90-min incubation period was selected for the standard assay to allow sufficient hydrolysis of substrate to detect liberated p-nitrophenol in specimens with low levels of enzyme activity. The lowest concentration of p-nitrophenol which could be reliably detected in our assay system was 12 nmoles.

The apparent K_m for β-galactosidases assayed at pH 3.6 was 2×10^{-4} M. The 2 mM substrate concentration selected for the standard assay theoretically provided sufficient substrate to saturate the system. At pH 6.5, the apparent K_m for the β-galactosidases in the enzyme preparation was 5×10^{-4} M. In the average assay, 0.3%–1% of the added substrate was hydrolized. The pH of the reaction mixture was examined at time zero and after 30 and 90 min of incubation at 37° C. The concentration of buffer used in the assay provided a stable pH throughout the pH range studied, which did not vary by

25

more than 0.1 pH unit after 90 min of incubation. The pH at which the enzymes were assayed did not alter the final development of yellow color at pH 10.7 in glycine-carbonate buffer.

The thermostability of the β-galactosidases in our enzyme preparations was not examined.

Electrophoresis

Vertical gel electrophoresis was performed on the supernatant obtained by centrifugation of the tissue homogenate using potato starch (Otto Hiller, Madison, Wis.) following the method of Smithies [12]. Citrate phosphate buffer was used for the electrode (0.04 M, pH 7.0) and for the gel (0.005 M, pH 7.2). Electrophoresis of enzyme samples was carried out for 16 hr at 160 v. The gel was removed and incubated with 4-methyl-umbelliferyl-β-D-galactopyranoside for 4 hr, then sprayed with a 0.2 M glycine-carbonate buffer, pH 10.7, and the areas of enzyme activity were located by their fluorescence under ultraviolet light.

STUDY PATIENTS

Control Patients

Hepatic tissue was obtained from six adults between the ages of 41 and 68 years undergoing abdominal surgery at Cleveland Metropolitan General Hospital for hiatal hernia, peptic ulcer, cholelithiasis, and, in one case, gastric tumor removal. None had metabolic disease. Two stillborns of 26- and 39-week gestations were analyzed approximately 90 min after delivery. The etiology of fetal wastage was not apparent in either case. It was not possible to examine matched control samples from normal children. Liver obtained within 1 hr after death from a 10-month-old male infant who died of sepsis and an 8-year-old female with degenerative brain disease of unknown etiology are included in the control group.

G_{M1} Gangliosidosis Patients

Early-onset patient. J. K. was a white male born after a full-term gestation to a 31-year-old gravida-4 mother. The infant was first hospitalized at age 3 months because of poor psychomotor development and enlargement of his liver and spleen. A female sibling died at 18 months with autopsy findings consistent with generalized gangliosidosis. Two other siblings are normal. During this child's first year, he showed evidence of retarded psychomotor development, hepatosplenomegaly, dysplastic changes in long bones and vertebra, and a cherry red spot in the macula.

Confirmatory laboratory data included vacuolated lymphocytes in peripheral blood smears and bone marrow, a rectal biopsy with PAS-positive material in ganglion cells, and diminished pH 3.6 β-galactosidase activity in leukocytes and cultured fibroblasts. Urines showed a normal concentration of dermatan and heparan sulfate, with no increase of keratan sulfate–like material. The child expired at age 18 months with autopsy findings identical to those described in other patients with this disease (E. Perrin, unpublished data). Liver tissue evaluated in this report was obtained at age $5\frac{1}{2}$ months under general anesthesia.

Late-onset patient. C. E. is a Negro male born after a 37-week gestation with a birth weight of 6 lb. Examination revealed left internal tibial torsion and metatarsus adductus which was treated with a cast for 7 months. Developmental guidelines appeared normal until 9–10 months of age. After this time, he slowly lost the ability to pull himself up, crawl, and transfer objects. At age 3 years, he showed severe spasticity and frequent seizures. He had no organomegaly, and the maculae were normal. Radiographically, there was early beaking of the lumbar vertebrae. Laboratory studies showed vacuolated lymphocytes in peripheral blood smears and bone marrow, glycolipid-containing ganglion cells on rectal biopsy, and markedly diminished β-galactosidase activity in urine, cultured skin fibroblasts, and white blood cells. The urine contained normal concentrations of dermatan and heparan sulfate, amino acids, and sulfatides. There was no increased excretion of keratan sulfate–like compounds in the urine. Cultured fibroblasts showed normal activities for aryl sulfatase A. At 32 months of age, an open liver biopsy was performed under local anesthesia.

RESULTS

Evidence for Variation in Hepatic Storage

Morphology. The liver of the early-onset case was enlarged and firm with a lobular appearance. Histologically, it showed a uniform panlobular change in which almost all parenchymal cells contained a cytoplasmic vacuole. The remaining cytoplasm was coarsely granular, almost foamy. The late-onset liver was grossly normal and histologically showed only a few vacuolated hepatocytes with scattered lymphocytic infiltrates in the portal tracts.

Electron micrographs of liver tissue from the early-onset type 1 patient showed that the majority of hepatocytes and Kupfer cells contained large empty intracytoplasmic vacuoles bounded by a single membrane. In marked contrast, the majority of the hepatic cells from the late-onset type 2 patient were normal, with a small amount of storage in Kupfer cells. The findings support quantitative rather than qualitative differences in cellular storage. The histological and electron-microscopic analyses of the liver tissue from both patients will be reported in detail in a separate publication (M. Petrelli and J. Blair, personal communication).

Chemical composition. Compositional analysis was performed by Dr. Kunihiko Suzuki according to methods previously described [13]. Results in table 1 show

TABLE 1

GANGLIOSIDE N-ACETYLNEURAMINIC ACID AND NONLIPID HEXOSAMINE IN LIVER

	Normal	Early Onset (Type 1)	Late Onset (Type 2)
N-acetylneuraminic acid	22	80	20
Nonlipid hexosamine	500	3,710	475

NOTE.—Values expressed as micrograms per 100 mg of chloroform-methanol insoluble residue. Analyses carried out by Dr. K. Suzuki.

that the liver from the type 1 patient contained an increased amount of ganglioside N-acetylneuraminic acid (a measure of G_{M1} ganglioside), in addition to a sevenfold elevation of nonlipid hexosamine, which reflects the concentration of the keratan sulfate–like material. In contrast, the late-onset liver showed no detectable excess of G_{M1} ganglioside and normal concentrations of nonlipid hexosamine.

Liver β-galactosidase activity. Figure 1 compares pH activity curves for β-galactosidase in liver from a normal adult, two stillborn infants, and the type 1 early-onset and type 2 late-onset patients. Normal adult liver showed a bell-shaped

27

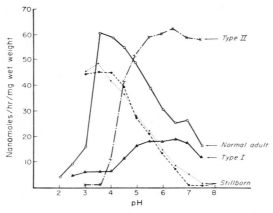

Fig. 1.—The pH-activity curves for β-galactosidase in supernatants obtained from liver homogenates (34,000 g).

activity curve with a pH optimum between 3.6 and 4.5, with decreasing activity as the hydrogen ion concentration was decreased. Fetal liver showed a similar pattern with a pH optimum between 3.6 and 4 but with less total activity than the adult liver at all pH's. The G_{M1} gangliosidosis patients showed similar patterns of activity which differed from the controls. Both patients had a depression of activity at pH 3.6–4, with maximal activity between pH 6 and 7.

Table 2 gives numerical comparisons of enzyme activity at pH 3.6 and 6.5 in all

TABLE 2

LIVER β-GALACTOSIDASE

| | | pH 3.6 | | pH 6.5 | |
	No. Studied	Mean	Range	Mean	Range
Control patients	8	45	19–61	22	13–30
Stillborn infants	2	...	45, 48	...	7, 8
G_{M1} patients:					
Type 1	J. K. 6	...		19	...
Type 2	C. E. 2	...		62	...

NOTE.—Values expressed as nanomoles per hour per milligram wet weight.

specimens studied. Both G_{M1} gangliosidosis patients showed deficient enzyme activity at pH 3.6. At pH 6.5, the early-onset type 1 patient had β-galactosidase activity within the range found for control patients, whereas the late-onset type 2 patient showed a significant increase in activity over control values. These patterns of activity did not change when the data were expressed in terms of solubilized supernatant protein.

Starch-Gel Electrophoresis

Starch-gel electrophoresis of supernatants obtained from liver homogenates and incubated with 4-methylumbelliferyl-β-D-galactopyranoside are shown in figure 2.

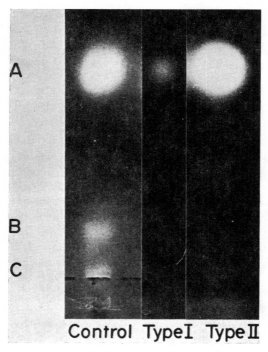

FIG. 2.—Starch-gel electrophoresis of supernatants obtained from liver homogenates (34,000 g). A 50-μg sample of protein was applied to each gel slot. Composite of separate electrophoreses.

A 50 μg sample of protein from the enzyme preparation was placed in each slot of the gel. Normal adult liver showed two slow-moving components near the origin (B and C) and one rapidly moving component (A). Incubation with 4-methylumbelliferyl-β-D-glucopyranoside showed one intense spot with a migration identical to the β-galactosidase A component. These results corroborate previously published results by Ho and O'Brien [14]. Electrophoresis of the 26-week stillborn liver differed from the eight controls studied in that no rapidly moving β-galactosidase was identified; however, a large spot was present after incubation with 4-methylumbelliferyl glucopyranoside.

The G_{M1} patients showed identical electrophoretic patterns. With 4-methylumbelliferyl-β-D-galactopyranoside, each showed a complete absence of the two slow-moving B and C components and the presence of a single rapidly moving A component. The increased intensity of the rapidly moving A enzyme in the type 2 liver correlated with the increased activity at pH 6.5. Incubation with 4-methyl-umbelliferyl-β-D-glucopyranoside demonstrated the presence of a single intense fluorescent spot with the same mobility as the rapidly moving β-galactosidase (A) enzyme in both G_{M1} patients.

DISCUSSION

Ho and O'Brien [14] and Öckerman and Hultberg [15] showed bell-shaped pH activity curves for normal human liver β-galactosidase similar to our data. This type of activity curve represents a composite of the activity of at least three forms of this enzyme. Two of the β-galactosidases separable by gel filtration have pH optima below pH 5 and correspond to the slow-moving B and C components on starch-gel electrophoresis; the third has maximal activity above pH 5 and corresponds to the rapidly moving A enzyme resolved by starch-gel electrophoresis [14, 15].

Both patients in this study showed maximal enzyme activity at pH 6–7, with a striking depression of activity at pH 3.6–4. In the early-onset type 1 patient, enzyme activity at pH 6.5 was comparable to normal controls, while the late-onset patient showed a tenfold increase of activity over control values. O'Brien et al. reported nearly normal activity for the pH 6.5 β-galactosidase in a type 2 patient but did not find pH 6.5 activity in type 1 patients [16]. This discrepancy may reflect the fact that their analyses on two type 1 patients were carried out on enzyme solubilized with water from liver tissue obtained at necropsy and stored frozen for variable periods, while our analyses were carried out immediately after liver biopsy on tissue hemogenates in which the enzyme was solubilized with detergent (J. S. O'Brien, personal communication).

Starch-gel electrophoresis of β-galactosidase from normal livers in this study showed two slow-moving components (B and C) near the origin and one rapidly moving component (A) confirming previous reports. O'Brien has reported that both types of G_{M1} gangliosidosis have complete absence of the slow-moving components B and C, with a rapidly moving A component persisting only in his late-onset type 2 patient. He suggested that two types of G_{M1} gangliosidosis could be defined, based on the presence or absence of the rapidly moving A enzyme [17]. In all patients reported to date, the B and C enzymes have been deficient. This was confirmed again in our two patients. However, the rapidly moving A component was definitely present in our early-onset type 1 child. Suzuki et al. have found the A enzyme in another child who was phenotypically type 1 [3]. We conclude from these data that the patterns of enzyme activity obtained by starch-gel electrophoresis or by pH activity curves cannot be used as a basis for classification, since type 1 as well as type 2 patients may show persistence of the A enzyme.

The polysaccharide stored in visceral organs and excreted in the urine of some patients represents an ill-defined polymer containing sialic acid, galactose, and glucosamine. Chemically, its composition resembles an undersulfated keratan sul-

15. ÖCKERMAN PA, HULTBERG B: Fractionation of 4-methylumbelliferyl-β-galactosidase activities in liver in gargoylism. *Scand J Clin Lab Invest* 22:199–202, 1968
16. O'BRIEN JS, OKADA S, Ho MW, et al: *Ganglioside Storage Disease in Lipid Storage Disease*. New York, Academic, 1970, pp 225–273
17. O'BRIEN JS: Five gangliosidoses. *Lancet* 2:805, 1969
18. CALLAHAN JW, WOLFE LS: Isolation and characterization of keratan sulfates from the liver of a patient with G_{M1} gangliosidosis type I. *Biochim Biophys Acta* 215: 527–543, 1970
19. PINSKY L, POWELL E, CALLAHAN J: G_{M1} gangliosidosis types I and II: enzymatic differences in cultured fibroblasts. *Nature* 228:1093–1095, 1970
20. Ho MW, O'BRIEN JS: Differential effect of chloride ions on β-galactosidase isoenzymes: a method for separate assay. *Clin Chim Acta* 32:443–450, 1971
21. JUNGALWALA FB, ROBINS E: Glycosidases in the nervous system. III. Separation, purification and substrate specificities of β-galactosidases and β-glucuronidase from brain. *J Biol Chem* 243:4258–4266, 1968
22. ROBINSON D, PRICE RG, DANCE N: Separation and properties of β-galactosidase, β-glucosidase, β-glucuronidase and N-acetyl-β-glucosaminidase from rat kidneys. *Biochem J* 102:525–532, 1967

Mucopolysaccharide Disorders

Sanfilippo Syndrome: Profound Deficiency of Alpha-Acetylglucosaminidase Activity in Organs and Skin Fibroblasts from Type-B Patients

JOHN S. O'BRIEN

The Sanfilippo syndrome is an inborn error of mucopolysaccharide metabolism characterized by severe progressive mental retardation, bony deformities, and excessive urinary excretion of heparan sulphate. The disorder is clinically distinct from related hereditary mucopolysaccharide storage diseases, such as Hurler's and Hunter's syndromes, and has been categorized as mucopolysaccharidosis Type 3 by Mc-Kusick (1). Analyses of pedigrees indicate that the disorder is transmitted as an autosomal recessive trait.

Kresse *et al.* (2) have demonstrated an impaired rate of degradation of acid mucopolysaccharides in cultured skin fibroblasts from patients with Sanfilippo syndrome. The defect in degradation can be corrected by addition of a macromolecular factor (corrective factor) to cultures of cells from patients with this disease. Corrective factor occurs in medium in which normal skin fibroblasts have been grown, and also in human urine.

Sanfilippo fibroblasts can be subclassified into two types, based on deficiencies of two different corrective factors (2). Fibroblasts from Sanfilippo Type A secrete a factor into the medium that corrects the abnormality of mucopolysaccharide degradation in fibroblasts from Sanfilippo Type-B patients

36

and vice versa. The two types of factor have been partially characterized; they are probably proteins with molecular weights of about 200,000, possessing different thermostability characteristics and different ionic charges at pH 8.5 (2).

I report here that activity of the lysosomal glycohydrolase α-acetylglucosaminidase (α-2-acetamido-2-deoxy-D-glucoside acetamidodeoxyglucohydrolase, EC 3.2.1.X, α-acetylglucosaminidase) is nearly absent in frozen organs and in cultured skin fibroblasts from patients with Type-B Sanfilippo syndrome.

MATERIALS AND METHODS

Kidney tissue was available from one patient with Sanfilippo syndrome; liver tissue was available from this patient and two others. Unfortunately, fibroblasts were not available from these three patients, and they were not classified as Sanfilippo Type A or B. Thus far, there are no evident clinical distinguishing features between Type-A and Type-B syndromes. One of these patients has been presented in detail as the prototype of Sanfilippo syndrome by McKusick (1). Frozen organs from patients with various other mucopolysaccharide storage diseases were also available. Tissues from controls and patients were stored frozen for periods of 2 months to 5 years before assay.

Skin fibroblast cultures were obtained from eight Sanfilippo patients, three with Type A, two with Type B, and three not subclassified. The subclassifications were made in the laboratory of Dr. Elizabeth Neufeld, National Institute of Health, Bethesda, Md. Fibroblast cultures from patients with other mucopolysaccharidoses were also available, as well as from parents of one of the patients.

All fibroblast cultures were grown as described (3–5), and were subcultured at least once before enzyme assay. Control fibroblast cultures were obtained from clinically normal children and adults of both sexes. Amniotic fluid cell cultures were taken from women undergoing amniocentesis during midpregnancy; they were selected from subjects in which a phenotypically normal baby was delivered. Lysosomal hydrolase enzyme activities increase progressively with time after subculture (4). Unless otherwise stated, enzyme assays were made 14 days after subculture; subcultures were begun at similar cell densities.

Fibroblast pellets were obtained by scraping cells from culture flasks, centrifuging at 3000 $\times$ g for 10 min, aspirating the supernatant medium, suspending the pellet in 0.95 M NaCl, centrifuging, aspirating the supernatant saline solution, and freezing the cell pellet at $-20°$ for 1 day to 3 weeks

37

before enzyme assay.

β-Galactosidase, β-acetylglucosaminidase, β-glucuronidase, β-glucosidase, α-galactosidase, and α-mannosidase were assayed in liver and fibroblast cultures with 4-methylumbelliferyl substrates (3–5).

Assay of p-nitrophenyl-α-L-fucosidase activity in fibroblast cultures was as follows. The cell pellet was weighed and homogenized in 5 volumes of distilled water in a ground-glass homogenizer. To 20 μl of homogenate was added 50 μl of p-nitrophenyl-α-L-fucopyranoside (1.5 mM in citrate–phosphate buffer, 0.1 M, pH 5.8), and the sample was incubated at 37° for 2 and 4 hr. The released p-nitrophenol was estimated as described below for assay of α-acetylglucosaminidase.

Assay of α-acetylglucosaminidase in liver, kidney, and cultured fibroblast pellets was as follows. The tissue or pellet was weighed and homogenized in 5 volumes of distilled water in a ground-glass homogenizer. To 20 μl of homogenate was added 50 μl of p-nitrophenyl-α-D-N-acetylglucosaminide (1.0 mM in citrate–phosphate buffer, pH 4.5, 0.1 M with respect to phosphate), and the sample was incubated at 37° for 2 and 4 hr. The reaction was stopped by addition of 100 μl of 3% trichloroacetic acid, after which it was centrifuged at 3000 × g for 10 min. The supernatant was then aspirated, taking care not to disturb the sediment; 350 μl of glycine–carbonate buffer (0.25 M, pH 10) was added to the supernatant, and absorbance was read at 420 nm on a spectrophotometer. Tissue blanks for each sample were prepared in the same manner, with distilled water substituted for the substrate. Final absorbances were obtained by subtraction of tissue-blank readings from sample readings.

A pH–activity curve was determined for α-acetylglucosaminidase in human liver tissue by the use of homogenates prepared as above; however, the final pH of the homogenate was varied between 3.5 and 7.0 with citrate–phosphate buffers (0.1–0.2 M). The pH optimum of the enzyme in liver and cultured fibroblasts was 4.5. Under the conditions described, activity of α-acetylglucosaminidase was linear over 4 hr of incubation. When the homogenate dilution was varied, the activity was not linear. Weissmann et al. (6) have described similar results in studies of α-acetylglucosaminidase from pig liver; they attribute the nonlinearity to endogenous inhibitors, which they could precipitate with ammonium sulfate.

When homogenate protein concentrations were kept constant from one sample to another by maintaining the same ratio of tissue wet weight to homogenate diluent (1:5), assays of duplicates agreed within ±10%. I did not attempt to optimize the concentration of p-nitrophenyl-α-D-N-acetylglucosaminide, due to the limited quantities of substrate available.

RESULTS

In frozen liver tissue from two patients with Sanfilippo syndrome, activities of α-acetylglucosaminidase were less than 10% of normal. A similar diminution was found in the kidney

TABLE 1.   *Alpha-acetylglucosaminidase in frozen organs*

Subjects	α-Acetylglucosaminidase
Liver	
Controls (13)	3.4
	(1.8–6.3)
Mucopolysaccharidoses	
Hurler's	37.0
Hurler's	27.0
Hunter's	3.7
Sanfilippo (D.F.)*	0.4
Sanfilippo(W.S.)*	0.3
Sanfilippo(C.L.)*	13.0
Kidney	
Controls (2)	3.9, 9.6
Sanfilippo (D.F.)	0.2

Enzyme activities are expressed as nmol of p-nitrophenol cleaved per mg of protein per hr at 37°.   Average and range of control values are given: numbers of controls studied are in parentheses.

* Patients were not classified as to Type A or Type B. For description of D. F. see (1).

of one of these patients. Elevated activity of α-acetylglucosaminidase was present in the liver tissue from one Sanfilippo patient (Table 1).

When liver homogenates from two patients were mixed in equal proportions with those from controls or with those from patients with other mucopolysaccharidoses, the activities of α-acetylglucosaminidase were the average of the two starting homogenates. These results indicated that soluble endogenous inhibitors did not account for the profound reduction of α-acetylglucosaminidase in the two patients tested. The activity of α-acetylglucosaminidase was not diminished in liver tissue from patients with Hurler's and Hunter's diseases (nor from one Sanfilippo patient), indicating that mucopolysaccharide storage *per se* was not responsible for the deficiency of α-acetylglucosaminidase activity.

39

TABLE 2. *Enzymatic activities in cultured skin fibroblasts*

Subjects	α-Acetyl-glucos-aminidase (A)	α-Fucosidase (B)	Ratio B/A
Controls (17)	5.4	18.4	3.4
	(2.1–12.6)	(2.3–41.9)	(2.0–6.3)
Mother of P.L.	2.4	26	10.6
Father of P.L.	2.8	34	12.1
Mucopolysaccharidoses			
Sanfilippo			
Type B (P.L.)	0.07	21	300
Type B (S.)	0.07	9	130
Type A (S.P.)	6.6	47	
Type A (M.P.)	7.2	52	
Type A (R.N.)	3.9	28	
Average and (range)	5.9(3.9–7.2)	42(28–52)	7
Unclassified (M-1)	3.4	11	
Unclassified (M-2)	2.7	9	
Unclassified (A.J.)	4.5	32	
Average and (range)	3.5(2.7–4.5)	17(9–32)	5
Hurler's	4.1	19	
Hunter's	4.5	16	
Hunter's	2.7	9	
Hunter's	5.3	22	
Average and (range)	4.2(2.7–4.5)	16(9–22)	4
Amniotic cultures (from normal pregnancies) (6)	4.6	55	12
	(1.7–9.4)	(35–74, 3 cases)	

Enzyme activities are expressed as nmol of p-nitrophenol cleaved per mg of protein per hr at 37°. Average and range of control values are given; numbers of cases studied are in parentheses.

Activities of β-acetylglucosaminidase, β-glucuronidase, β-glucosidase, α-galactosidase, and α-mannosidase were either normal or elevated in liver tissue from the Sanfilippo patients. Activities of β-galactosidase were reduced to 30–50% of control values in all patients with mucopolysaccharide storage diseases.

α-Acetylglucosaminidase activity in fibroblast cultures from two Type-B Sanfilippo patients was barely detectable; values were less than 0.07 nmol cleaved per mg of protein per hr. A more sensitive assay technique will be necessary to find whether any α-acetylglucosaminidase activity is present in fibroblasts from such patients.

In one experiment, α-acetylglucosaminidase was assayed in fibroblasts from a single patient at 10, 14, and 21 days after subculture; the same degree of deficiency was found at each time. The deficiency of α-acetylglucosaminidase was present in cultures from the same patient, grown over a 3-month period (more than 10 cell generations). Mixture of fibroblast homogenates from controls (including those with Type-A Sanfilippo syndrome with those from Type-B Sanfilippo patients demonstrated that soluble endogenous inhibitors did not account for the striking deficiency of α-acetylglucosaminidase activity.

Activities of β-galactosidase, β-acetylglucosaminidase, β-glucuronidase, β-glucosidase, α-galactosidase, α-mannosidase, and α-fucosidase were within the normal range in fibroblasts from Type-B patients. No deficiency of α-acetylglucosaminidase activity was present in fibroblasts from patients with other mucopolysaccharidoses, including those with Type-A Sanfilippo (Table 2).

The specific activities of α-acetylglucosaminidase in cultured fibroblasts from both parents of one patient were in the low-normal range (Table 2). When ratios of α-acetylglucosaminidase to α-fucosidase activities were calculated, they were abnormally high (Table 2), indicating a deficiency of α-acetylglucosaminidase relative to α-fucosidase in cells from the heterozygous parents.

α-Acetylglucosaminidase activity was readily demonstrated in amniotic fluid cells, at levels similar to those found in cultured skin fibroblasts (Table 2). α-Fucosidase activity was higher in amniotic cells than in skin fibroblasts.

DISCUSSION

The data suggest that a deficiency of α-acetylglucosaminidase* is the primary enzyme defect in Type-B Sanfilippo syndrome. The defect is specific for α-acetylglucosaminidase. The

---

* Recently, I have found that the activity of α-acetylglucosaminidase with phenyl-α-D-N-acetylglucosaminide as substrate is also markedly diminished in tissues from patients with Type-B Sanfilippo syndrome.

enzyme is a lysosomal glycohydrolase, distinctly different from β-acetylglucosaminidase, α- and β-glucosidase, α-mannosidase, β-glucuronidase, α-L-fucosidase, β-D-xylosidase, α-acetylgalactosaminidase (6), and hyaluronidase (7). The defect persists over many cell generations. The enzyme is partially deficient in cells from obligate heterozygotes. The mucopolysaccharide that accumulates in Sanfilippo syndrome possesses α-linked N-acetylglucosamine residues (8), and appears to be stored in lysosomes (9). The deficiency of a lysosomal degradative enzyme, probably involved in heparan sulfate degradation, fits well with the impairment of mucopolysaccharide degradation (2) in cells from patients with Type-B Sanfilippo syndrome.

The Type-B correction factor is probably identical to α-acetylglucosaminidase. This factor, isolated from human urine, is destroyed by heating to 70° in 0.95 N NaCl for 10 min (2). In homogenates of cultured skin fibroblasts, prepared as described for assay above, I have found that the activity of α-acetylglucosaminidase is destroyed by heating at 70° for 10 min. If α-acetylglucosaminidase and Type-B correction factor are identical, the purified enzyme may prove to have clinical utility.

Recently, Kresse and Neufeld (10) have purified the Type-A corrective factor 850-fold from normal human urine, and have shown it to possess no α-acetylglucosaminidase activity, emphasizing again the genotype specificity of the two types of Sanfilippo syndrome. The Type-A corrective factor appears to be a heparan sulfate sulfatase (10).

The fact that activity for α-acetylglucosaminidase is present in normal amniotic fluid cells taken in midpregnancy indicates that Type-B Sanfilippo syndrome, a fatal hereditary disorder with a 25% recurrence risk, may be diagnosed prenatally by amniocentesis and enzyme assay, in the same manner as is now used for Tay-Sachs disease (11).

I thank Prof. Bernard Weissmann for generous gifts of phenyl- and p-nitrophenyl-α-D-N-acetylglucosaminides used as substrates. Frozen tissues and fibroblast cultures from the patients studied here were supplied by Drs. C. I. Scott, A. Crocker, A. Fluharty, H. Kihara, R. Matalon, C. R. Scott, and E. F. Neufeld. Technical assistance was provided by Mrs. M. L. Veath and L. Tennant. This work was supported by grants from the National Foundation–March of Dimes, The National Genetics Foundation, and National Institute of Health Grants NS-08682 and GM-17702 (Program Project).

1. McKusick, V. A. (1966) in *Heritable Disorders of Connective Tissue* (C. V. Mosby Co., St. Louis), 357–361.
2. Kresse, H., Wiesmann, U., Cantz, M., Hall, C. W. & Neufeld, E. F. (1971) *Biochem. Biophys. Res. Commun.* **42**, 892–898.

3. Ho, M. W., Seck, J., Schmidt, D., Veath, M. L., Johnson, W., Brady, R. O. & O'Brien, J. S. (1972) *Amer. J. Hum. Genet.* **24**, 37–45.

4. Okada, S., Veath, M. L., Leroy, J. & O'Brien, J. S. (1971) *Amer. J. Hum. Genet.* **23**, 55–61.

5. Leroy, J. G., Ho, M. W., MacBrinn, M. C., Zielke, K., Jacob, J. & O'Brien, J. S. (1972) *Pediat. Res.*, in press.

6. Weissmann, B., Rowin, G., Marshall, J. & Friederici, D. (1967) *Biochemistry* **6**, 207–214.

7. Roseman, S. & Dorfman, A. (1951) *J. Biol. Chem.* **191**, 607–620.

8. For a review, see Dorfman, A. & Matalon, R. (1972) in *Metabolic Basis of Inherited Disease*, eds Stanbury, J. B., Wyngaarten, J. B. & Frederickson, D. F. (McGraw-Hill, New York, 3rd ed., chap. 49.

9. Dodion, J., Résibois, A., Loeb, H. & Crémer, N. (1966) *Pathol. Eur.* **1**, 50–66.

10. Kresse, H. & Neufeld, E. (1972) *J. Biol. Chem.*, **247**, 2164–2170.

11. O'Brien, J. S., Okada, S., Fillerup, D. L., Veath, M. L., Adornato, B., Brenner, P. & Lreoy, J. (1971) *Science* **172**, 61–64.

Classification of the Mucopolysaccharidoses Based on the Pattern of Mucopolysacchariduria

DAVID KAPLAN, M.D.

SINCE the original description of the Hurler syndrome [1] and appreciation that this disease was characterized by excretion of excessive amounts of heparan sulfate and dermatan sulfate in the urine [2–4], it has become apparent that there are actually several syndromes, clinically similar, in which patients excrete either heparan sulfate or dermatan sulfate, or excrete both in varying proportions. In 1964 Terry and Linker [5], studying six patients of their own and reviewing the literature, thought that they could distinguish four discrete syndromes based on the pattern of urinary mucopolysaccharide excretion. Subsequently, on the basis of clinical criteria, a classification into five groups was proposed, namely, mucopolysaccharidoses types I, II, III, V and VI or, eponymically, the Hurler, Hunter, Sanfillipo, Scheie and Maroteaux-Lamy syndromes, respectively [6]. All these patients were found to excrete either heparan sulfate, dermatan sulfate or both in excessive quantities in the urine.

I propose to present data herein on the excessive urinary mucopolysaccharide excretion in forty-six patients and to use these data as a basis for classification. Four distinct patterns of mucopolysaccharide excretion were found*: (1) heparan sulfate excretors, (2) dermatan sulfate excretors, (3) excretors of both heparan sulfate and dermatan sulfate in approximately equal proportions and (4) excretors

*Excretors of keratan sulfate (the Morquio syndrome) were not included; they were described previously [7].

of both with a predominance of dermatan sulfate. Correlations were then made between these four patterns of mucopolysaccharide excretion and the major clinical findings present in the mucopolysaccharide storage diseases: mental retardation, aortic ring or valve disease, corneal opacification, hepatomegaly, splenomegaly and skeletal abnormalities. There was an apparent correlation between certain clinical abnormalities and the type of mucopolysaccharide found in the urine.

MATERIALS AND METHODS

Urine preserved with a small amount of chloroform was obtained from patients suspected of having mucopolysaccharide storage diseases throughout the United States, Canada and the United Kingdom. For transit times greater than twenty-four hours the urine was shipped refrigerated or frozen. Upon arrival, the urine was refrigerated for twenty-four hours, the supernatant separated from the precipitated salts, diluted with a half volume of distilled water, brought to pH 5.0 with glacial acetic acid and refrigerated overnight after the addition of one thirtieth volume of 2.5 per cent aqueous cetylpyridinium chloride. The resulting precipitate was washed in sodium chloride saturated 95 per cent ethanol, dissolved in a small amount of 5 per cent sodium acetate, 0.5 N acetic acid, stirred with chloroform and amyl alcohol (3:1 mixture), and, after separation by centrifugation, the aqueous phase was reprecipitated with three volumes of 95 per cent ethanol and refrigerated overnight. The precipitate was washed in 80 per cent ethanol, redissolved in the acetate buffer and stirred with Lloyd's reagent and kaolin (2:1 mixture), and the mucopolysaccharide was again precipitated with ethanol. The precipitate was dissolved in distilled water, retreated with Lloyd's reagent and kaolin, and the purified mucopolysaccharide fractionally was precipitated as the calcium salt with ethanol, dried and weighed.

The following analyses were performed for each fraction: the carbazole and orcinol reactions for uronic acid [8,9], the anthrone reaction for neutral sugar [10] and separation and quantitation of the amino sugars by column chromatography [7]. In addition, on appropriate samples the following analyses were also made: paper chromatography for galactose [11] and L-iduronic acid [12], optical rotation, digestion with testicular hyaluronidase [13] and sulfate analysis [14].

Estimation of the relative amounts of heparan sulfate and dermatan sulfate in a urine specimen which appeared to contain significant quantities of both gave the most difficulty in these analyses. These two substances could not be satisfactorily

separated by column chromatography using cellulose [15], ECTEOLA cellulose [16] or DEAE Sephadex® [17], when the urinary mucopolysaccharide was added either free or as a cetylpyridinium complex and eluted with increasing salt concentrations by either stepwise or gradient elution. However, these methods also failed to separate authentic heparan sulfate and dermatan sulfate from urine when they were added to normal urine and subjected to chromatography. The presumed mixture of heparan sulfate and dermatan sulfate was therefore subjected to treatment with testicular hyaluronidase and the undigested mucopolysaccharide was reisolated and treated with alkaline copper [18] to separate dermatan sulfate from heparan sulfate. This method did permit crude quantitation of the relative amounts of the two mucopolysaccharides and the results showed good agreement with the relative amounts of glucosamine and galactosamine in these samples.

Clinical data from patients not personally seen were obtained from the physicians who supplied the urine samples, usually in the form of abstracts of hospital admissions which often included photographs and roentgenograms.

RESULTS

As noted earlier, on the basis of the urinary findings the patients could be divided into four groups. Typical results are presented of analyses of urinary mucopolysaccharides of two subjects in each group, followed by a summary table for each group containing the pertinent clinical and biochemical data.

Heparansulfaturia. In Table I are shown the results of two analyses of urine. Several things are apparent: (1) the carbazole to orcinol ratios are high (1.6 and 2.4), (2) the predominant hexosamine is glucosamine (93 per cent and 68 per cent), (3) L-iduronic acid is not demonstrable on the paper chromatograms, (4) a high positive optical rotation is demonstrated on the one sample tested, (5) only minimal quantities of galactose are present, and (6) in one sample, the percentage of mucopolysaccharide lost after treatment with testicular hyaluronidase is approximately equal to the percentage of galactosamine in the sample. Such data suggest that the major component of the urinary mucopolysaccharide in these two patients is heparan sulfate, that the remainder is predominantly chondroitin sulfate A or C and that minimal amounts of dermatan sulfate and keratan sulfate are present.

TABLE I
ANALYSES OF URINARY MUCOPOLYSACCHARIDE FROM TWO SUBJECTS

Alc. Fx. (%)	Weight (kg.)	Carbazole (%)	Orcinol (%)	Anthrone (%)	GluNH$_2$:GalNH$_2$	
		*Subject 6: fifteen year old girl, 1,320 ml. of urine*				
28	23.8	27.8	18.1	5.3	92:8	No L-iduronic acid
33	50.5	36.5	20.7	5.3	96:4	...
41	54.6	45.4	27.3	7.3	91:9	$[\alpha]^{23°}$D = +58
45	12.6	33.8	23.0	8.2	90:10	...
64	35.2	27.5	18.4	8.1	91:9	Galactose: ±
Mean	...	36.1	22.1	...	93:7	...
		Total mucopolysaccharide = 134 mg./L.; carbazole:orcinol = 1.63				
		*Subject 2: ten year old boy, 1,240 ml. of urine*				
28	42.5	37.8	19.3	7.9	88:12	No L-iduronic acid
37	66.9	39.6	11.1	6.6	67:33	...
45	42.3	32.8	17.7	7.6	44:56	60% loss after hyaluronidase
64	17.7	28.8	15.5	9.7	78:22	Galactose: 1+
Mean	...	36.3	15.2	...	68:32	...
		Total mucopolysaccharide = 136 mg./L.; carbazole:orcinol = 2.39				

NOTE: Alc. Fx. and Weight = milligrams of mucopolysaccharide precipitated at designated ethanol concentration. GluNH$_2$:GalNH$_2$ = ratio of glucosamine to galactosamine. L-iduronic acid and galactose estimated by paper chromatography after hydrolysis. Loss after hyaluronidase refers to percentage of substrate not recoverable after treatment with testicular hyaluronidase.

Table II summarizes the results in fifteen patients with similar patterns of urinary mucopolysaccharide excretion, including two patients who were studied on more than one occasion. The mean mucopolysaccharide excretion is 131 mg. per L., the normal in our laboratory being 5 to 25 mg. per L. The major amino sugar is glucosamine; in normal urinary mucopolysaccharide the major amino sugar is galactosamine because heparan sulfate and keratan sulfate are present in only trace amounts [7,19,20].

TABLE II
SUMMARY OF LABORATORY AND CLINICAL DATA ON FIFTEEN HEPARAN SULFATE EXCRETORS*

Subject	Age (yr.) and Sex	MPS (mg./L.)	GluNH$_2$: GalNH$_2$	Carbazole: Orcinol	Mental Retardation	Aortic Disease	Corneal Opacities	Hepatomegaly	Splenomegaly	Skeletal Changes
1	10,M	93	86:14	2.55	+	−	−	−	−	+
2	9,M	205	72:28	1.71	+	−	−	+	−	+
	10	136	68:32	2.55						
3	4,M	59	84:16	1.74	+	−	−	+	−	+
4	6,M	124	80:20	2.93	+	−	−	+	−	+
5	11,M	120	73:27	2.30	+	−	−	+	+	+
6	15,F	120	84:16	1.77	+	−	−	+	−	+
	16	134	93:7	1.63						
7	2,F	107	78:22	2.92	+	...	−	+	−	+
8	2,F	148	91:9	2.26	+	−	−	+	+	+
9	10,F	123	88:12	3.14	+	−	−	−	−	+
10	5,M	225	90:10	3.39	+	−	−	+	+	+
11	4,F	264	87:13	3.12	+	−	−	+	−	+
12	1,M	118	91:9	1.67	−	−	−	−	−	+
13	3,F	99	89:11	1.82	−	−	−	+	+	+
14	10,M	64	82:18	1.64	+	−	−	−	−	+
15	2,F	95	85:15	2.40	+	−	−	+	−	+

* Eight male and seven female; mean age six years. MPS = mucopolysaccharide. GluNH$_2$:GalNH$_2$ and Carbazole:Orcinol as in Table I. The + and − signs indicate the presence or absence of the indicated clinical findings.

TABLE III

ANALYSES OF URINARY MUCOPOLYSACCHARIDE FROM TWO SUBJECTS

Alc. Fx. (%)	Weight (kg.)	Carbazole (%)	Orcinol (%)	Anthrone (%)	GluNH₂: GalNH₂	L-Iduronic Acid	% Sensitive to Hyaluronidase

Subject 16: one year old girl, 830 ml. of urine							
23	69.4	13.9	34.4	4.9	2:98	4+	0
33	28.0	20.0	28.0	5.4	5:95	3+	10
37	20.5	15.3	24.1	7.5	9:91	3+	40
45	6.5	33.2	20.9	7.5	6:94	1+	...
64	25.9	28.4	19.6	8.8	9:91	0	90
Mean	...	18.5	28.4	...	5:95	...	~25
Total mucopolysaccharide = 181 mg./L.; carbazole:orcinol = 0.65							
Subject 21: seventeen year old girl, 675 ml. of urine							
23	75.0	14.8	50.4	6.8	5:95	4+	10
41	16.6	22.8	32.2	7.4	5:95	2+⎫	
47	9.8	22.2	27.7	7.8	2:98	1+⎬	50
64	15.5	17.2	45.7	19.0	14:86	2+⎭	
Mean	...	16.9	45.2	...	6:94	...	~25
Total mucopolysaccharide = 173 mg./L.; carbazole:orcinol = 0.37							

NOTE: First seven columns of data as in Table I. Last column indicates that after digestion with testicular hyaluronidase about 25 per cent of the mucopolysaccharide in both cases was digested and not recoverable.

Clinically, the fifteen patients with this type of mucopolysacchariduria form a homogeneous group. None of them has corneal opacification or detectable disease of the aorta. All but two are mentally retarded, and the two who are not are among the youngest and evidence of mental retardation may be expected to develop as they grow older [6]. These patients thus meet the criteria for the diagnosis of the Sanfillipo syndrome [21] or mucopolysaccharidosis, type III [6]. In several of the patients this syndrome could not be differentiated from one of the other variants of the mucopolysaccharide storage diseases, prior to characterization of the urinary mucopolysaccharide.

Dermatansulfaturia. Table III shows the results of two urinalyses in patients who are excretors of dermatan sulfate. The evidence for this conclusion is based on the following data: (1) the low carbazole to orcinol ratio (0.65 and 0.37), (2) the predominance of galactosamine and (3) the presence of L-iduronic acid. The absence of significant quantities of glucosamine precludes the presence of excess heparan sulfate, and since approximately 25 per cent of the mucopolysaccharide is degraded by testicular hyaluronidase, the presence of chondroitin sulfate A or C in amounts close to the normal range is indicated.

The laboratory and clinical data in this group of patients (Table IV) suggest that they

comprise a discrete group. The first four patients are siblings, as are patients 20 and 21, and patients 22 and 23. No patient is mentally retarded. All have corneal disease and six of the eight have evidence of aortic disease, either by auscultation or on chest roentgenogram. In the previous clinical classification system, then, they would be considered examples of the Maroteaux-Lamy syndrome [22] or mucopolysaccharidosis, type VI [6].

Mixed Mucopolysacchariduria, Type A. Table V contains examples of analyses of urine from patients who fall into the group of patients who excrete approximately equal proportions of heparan sulfate and dermatan sulfate. The analytic data differ clearly from values presented as examples of heparansulfaturia and dermatansulfaturia. Analysis of the 28 per cent ethanol fraction indicates a predominance of dermatan sulfate. The higher alcohol fractions show the major portion of the amino sugar to be glucosamine, and the alkaline copper method demonstrates the presence of significant quantities of heparan sulfate. The urines of twelve such subjects have been evaluated and the results are rather uniform. In the cases studied, the amounts of heparan sulfate and dermatan sulfate are approximately equal; this is confirmed by the hexosamine analyses, which gave a mean glucosamine to galactosamine ratio of 48:52. The

47

Subject	Age (yr.) and Sex	MPS (mg./L.)	GluNH₂: GalNH₂	Carbazole: Orcinol	Mental Retarda-tion	Aortic Disease	Corneal Opacities	Hepato-megaly	Spleno-megaly	Skeletal Changes
16	1,F	181	5:95	0.65	−	+	+	+	+	+
17	4,F	185	5:95	0.66	−	+	+	+	+	+
	7	62		0.49						
	8	56		0.49						
18	3,M	90	7:93	0.66	−	+	+	+	+	+
19	6,F	249	6:94	0.54	−	+	+	+	+	+
	10	95		0.44						
20	15,F	124	7:93	0.41	−	+	+	+	−	+
21	17,M	173	6:94	0.37	−	+	+	+	−	+
22	10,M	238	6:94	0.49	−	−	+	+	+	+
23	8,M	255	5:95	0.53	−	−	+	+	+	+

* Four male and four female; the mean age was eight years at time of the initial study. Abbreviations and symbols as in Table II.

most striking clinical finding is that all the patients are male and thus correspond to the sex-linked Hunter syndrome, or mucopoly-saccharidosis, type II [6]. Clinically, they are somewhat more closely allied to the patients with heparansulfaturia in that they are likely to be mentally retarded, only two of the twelve have corneal changes and none have detect-able aortic disease. In the opinion of the ob-servors submitting the urine samples, the pa-tients were considered to be examples of either the Hurler or Hunter syndrome. In accord with the current impression, the more severely

affected usually received the former designa-tion, and the less affected the latter.

Mixed Mucopolysacchariduria, Type B. The patterns of urinary mucopolysaccharide excretion characteristic of this group are shown in Table VII. As in the previous group, both heparan sulfate and dermatan sulfate are excreted in excess, but here there is a clear preponderance of dermatan sulfate. As in mixed mucopolysacchariduria, type A, the first (28 per cent) ethanol fraction appears to contain almost exclusively dermatan sulfate. Unlike mixed mucopolysacchariduria, type A,

TABLE V
ANALYSES OF URINARY MUCOPOLYSACCHARIDE IN TWO SUBJECTS

Alc. Fx. (%)	Weight (kg.)	Carbazole (%)	Orcinol (%)	Anthrone (%)	GluNH₂: GalNH₂	L-Iduronic Acid
Subject 28: ten year old boy, 1,040 ml. of urine						
28	55.4	13.3	38.2	5.3	15:85	4+
38	45.3	20.3	25.3	4.8	64:36	2+
45	39.3	20.2	20.8	5.3	58:42	±
64	37.1	18.8	20.7	6.0	70:30	0
Mean	...	17.8	27.4	...	48:52	
Total mucopolysaccharide = 170 mg./L.; carbazole:orcinol = 0.65						
Subject 27: five year old boy, 745 ml. of urine						
28	59.2	20.5	39.6	4.7	24:76	3+
45	64.0	38.8	27.5	7.1	60:40	1+
64	15.2	24.7	16.0	9.7	75:25	0
Mean	...	29.3	31.3	...	46:54	...
Total mucopolysaccharide = 186 mg./L.; carbazole:orcinol = 0.97						

NOTE: Ethanol fractions from patient 28 pooled and 50 mg. treated with testicular hyaluronidase, from which 39 mg. was recovered. Treatment with alkaline copper yielded 20 mg. of heparan sulfate and 19 mg. of dermatan sulfate (51:49). Similar treatment of patient 27 yielded 18 mg. of heparan sulfate and 19 mg. of dermatan sulfate (49:51).

TABLE VI

SUMMARY OF LABORATORY AND CLINICAL DATA ON TWELVE SUBJECTS WHO EXCRETED APPROXIMATELY EQUAL AMOUNTS OF HEPARAN SULFATE AND DERMATAN SULFATE

Subject	Age (yr.) and Sex	MPS (mg/L.)	GluNH₂: GalNH₂	Carbazole: Orcinol	HS:DS (est.)	Mental Retardation	Aortic Disease	Corneal Opacities	Hepatomegaly	Splenomegaly	Skeletal Changes
24	33,M	60	50:50	0.89	...	+	−	+	+	+	+
25	8,M	348	47:53	1.13	52:48	+	−	−	+	+	+
26	2,M	346	50:50	0.85	...	+	−	−	+	+	+
		173		0.82	...						
		236	46:54	0.85	...						
		169		0.85	...						
27	5,M	186	46:54	0.94	49:51	+	−	+	+	+	+
28	10,M	170	48:52	0.72	51:49	+	−	−	+	−	+
29	2,M	87	48:52	1.02	...	+	−	−	−	−	+
30	15,M	171	44:56	0.79	...	−	−	−	+	+	+
31	5,M	168	45:55	0.98	...	+	−	+	+	−	+
32	6,M	197	48:52	1.16	53:47	−	−	−	+	−	+
33	43,M	50	47:53	0.64	45:55	−	−	−	+	+	+
34	5,M	108	46:54	0.93	50:50	−	−	−	−	−	+
35	8,M	48	53:47	1.23	...	−	−	−	+	+	+

NOTE: Subject 26 was studied four times over a ten week period. HS:DS (est.) = the estimated proportions of heparan sulfate (HS) and dermatan sulfate (DS) in the urinary mucopolysaccharide.

this 28 per cent fraction makes up half or more of the total mucopolysaccharide isolated from these urines. From the higher alcohol fractions, heparan sulfate may be isolated after treatment with testicular hyaluronidase. Table VIII shows the results in eleven patients with similar analytic data. These results differ from those in Table VI: a higher proportion of dermatan sulfate and, as would be expected, a higher proportion of galactosamine is present compared to glucosamine. Table VIII demonstrates that there is two or three times as much dermatan sulfate as heparan sulfate and that the mean glucosamine to galactosamine ratio is 27:73. The same table also demonstrates that the patients are also somewhat different from those listed in Table VI in terms of clinical findings. In a sense, they complete the clinical spectrum—falling between the patients with dermatansulfaturia and those who excrete both dermatan sulfate and heparan sulfate in equal proportions. Clinical diagnoses of these patients included the Hurler syndrome, the Hunter syndrome,

TABLE VII

ANALYSES OF URINARY MUCOPOLYSACCHARIDES IN TWO SUBJECTS

Alc. Fx. (%)	Weight (kg.)	Carbazole (%)	Orcinol (%)	Anthrone (%)	GluNH₂: GalNH₂	L-Iduronic Acid
Subject 36: forty-seven year old man, 1,040 ml. of urine						
28	38.7	12.8	37.4	8 4	11:89	4+
38	13.0	20.9	30.6	6.7	46:54	2+
45	8.1	21.1	31.3	7.3	45:55	2+
64	5 5	17.2	23.1	7 6	39:61	1+
Mean	...	15.8	34.1	...	25:75	...
Total mucopolysaccharide = 63 mg./L.; carbazole:orcinol = 0.46						
Subject 37: thirty-four year old woman, 1,070 ml. of urine						
28	67.4	16.7	34.3	5.4	14:85	4+
38	25.9	25.4	30.2	5.7	52:48	2+
45	21.9	26.7	27.5	6.1	49:51	1+
64	24.6	21.8	18.1	7.7	40:60	0
Mean	...	20.8	29.6	...	24:76	...
Total mucopolysaccharide = 131 mg./L.; carbazole:orcinol = 0.70						

NOTE: Ethanol fractions from subject 37 pooled and 50 mg. treated with testicular hyaluronidase, from which 34 mg. was recovered. Treatment with alkaline copper yielded 10 mg. of heparan sulfate and 24 mg. of dermatan sulfate (29:71).

49

TABLE VIII

SUMMARY OF LABORATORY AND CLINICAL DATA ON ELEVEN SUBJECTS WHO EXCRETED TWO OR THREE TIMES AS MUCH DERMATAN SULFATE AS HEPARAN SULFATE[*]

Subject	Age (yr.) and Sex	MPS (mg./L.)	GluNH$_2$:GalNH$_2$	Carbazole:Orcinol	HS:DS (est.)	Mental Retardation	Aortic Disease	Corneal Opacities	Hepatomegaly	Splenomegaly	Skeletal Changes
36	47,M	58	...	0.61	...	−	+	+	+	+	+
	48	63	25:75	0.49	...						
	51	48	...	0.54	...						
37	34,F	131	24:76	0.70	29:71	−	+	+	+	−	+
38	9,M	245	24:76	0.58	30:70	+	−	+	+	−	+
39	7,M	258	27:73	0.56	32:68	+	−	−	+	+	+
40	32,M	75	35:65	0.70	...	−	+	+	−	−	+
41	30,F	52	32:68	0.67	...	−	+	+	−	−	+
42	7,F	152	23:77	0.46	...	−	+	+	+	+	+
	9	175	...	0.47	...						
43	2,M	83	33:67	0.54	...	+	−	+	+	+	+
44	4,M	178	35:65	0.76	25:75	−	−	−	+	−	+
45	6,F	86	22:78	0.55	...	+	−	+	+	+	+
46	2,M	229	23:77	0.65	30:70	+	−	+	+	+	+

* Seven male and four female; mean age sixteen years.

the Scheie syndrome and the "adult form" of the Hurler syndrome [5]. Patient 42 was considered at age seven to be an example of the Scheie syndrome and at age nine an example of the Hurler syndrome.

Repeat Studies. Nine patients were studied on more than one occasion (Tables II,·IV, VI and VIII). Except in one case, the results of study of the urinary mucopolysaccharide were not sufficiently changed from the first examination to justify reclassification of the patient.

Family Studies. Extensive studies were not carried out on the urine of family members of the propositi, but samples were obtained from the parents of subjects 2 and 6 (who were siblings), the mother and two clinically unaffected siblings of subject 15, and the mother of subjects 16 through 19. The urinary mucopolysaccharide excretion was normal in all cases. This finding is compatible with the results of one group of investigators [19], but not of another [23].

COMMENTS

It appears warranted to conclude that it would be better to classify the mucopolysaccharide storage diseases on the basis of the pattern of urinary mucopolysaccharide excretion rather than on clinical grounds. It is true that there is little difficulty in distinguishing patients at either end of the biochemical spectrum (heparan sulfate excretors from dermatan sulfate excretors) from one another on purely clinical grounds. However, there may be considerable difficulty in distinguishing these patients from patients with the Hurler, Hunter or Scheie syndrome, or distinguishing patients with one of these three syndromes from one another.

Indeed, on the basis of the urinary excretion of mucopolysaccharide, there are not five syndromes, but four. Assuming that one is able to attach the correct eponymic designation, the data suggest the following classification: Heparansulfaturia = the Sanfillipo syndrome or mucopolysaccharidosis, type III; dermatansulfaturia = the Maroteaux-Lamy syndrome or mucopolysaccharidosis, type VI; mixed mucopolysacchariduria, type A = the Hunter syndrome or mucopolysaccharidosis, type II; and mixed mucopolysacchariduria, type B = both the Hurler and the Scheie syndromes or mucopolysaccharidoses, types I and V. The clinical correlations with these four varieties of mucopolysacchariduria suggest that mental retardation is associated with the excretion of heparan sulfate and that corneal opacification and aortic disease are associated with the excretion of dermatan sulfate. When both are excreted, varying combinations of these three abnormalities are found. Skeletal changes of varying degree are found in patients with all four types, although this may partly reflect the type of patient selected for study. The presence or absence of hepatomegaly or splenomegaly is not helpful in differentiating one syndrome from another.

The second conclusion which may be drawn from these data is that determination of the glucosamine to galactosamine ratio of the iso-

TABLE IX

SUMMARY OF BIOCHEMICAL AND CLINICAL DATA FROM FORTY-SIX PATIENTS WITH MUCOPOLYSACCHARIDURIA

Type of Mucopolysacchariduria	No. of Subjects	Mean MPS (range)	Mean % GluNH$_2$ (range)	Mean % GalNH$_2$ (range)	Mean C:O (range)	Mental Retardation (%)	Aortic Disease (%)	Corneal Opacity (%)	Hepatomegaly (%)	Splenomegaly (%)	Skeletal Changes (%)	Previous Classifications [6]	
												Eponymic	Mucopolysaccharidosis
Heparansulfaturia	15	131 (59–264)	84 (68–93)	16 (7–32)	2.33 (1.63–3.39)	87	0	0	67	27	100	Sanfilippo	Type III
Mixed mucopolysacchariduria, type A	12	168 (48–348)	48 (44–53)	52 (47–56)	0.92 (0.64–1.23)	58	0	25	83	58	100	Hunter	Type II
Mixed mucopolysacchariduria, type B	11	131 (48–258)	28 (22–35)	72 (65–78)	0.59 (0.46–0.76)	45	45	82	73	45	100	Hurler and Scheie	Types I and V
Dermatansulfaturia	8	155 (56–255)	6 (5–7)	94 (93–95)	0.52 (0.37–0.66)	0	75	100	100	75	100	Maroteaux-Lamy	Type VI

NOTE: MPS = urinary mucopolysaccharide excretion in milligrams per liter. % GluNH$_2$ = per cent of mucopolysaccharide hexosamine that is glucosamine. % GalNH$_2$ = per cent of mucopolysaccharide hexosamine that is galactosamine. C:O = ratio of color development with carbazole reagent to color development with orcinol reagent (tests for uronic acid content of mucopolysaccharide).

lated mucopolysaccharide may be sufficient for classification. The total amounts of mucopolysaccharide per liter of urine do not differ from one group to another. The ratio of color development with carbazole and orcinol, although it differentiates the heparan sulfate excretors from the other three types, does not reliably differentiate these three syndromes from one another. As would be expected, however, the carbazole to orcinol ratio does tend to be lower in patients who excrete a greater proportion of dermatan sulfate.

Table IX summarizes the data which provide the basis for these two conclusions and appears to represent a reasonable scheme for the classification of the mucopolysaccharide storage disease.

The data provide minimal additional insight into the possible biochemical abnormalities responsible for these syndromes. Studies from several laboratories are compatible with either a failure of proper degradation or, more likely, a failure of normal synthesis of the protein-polysaccharide complex present in tissues. Dorfman [24] has previously noted that the heparan sulfate from the liver of a child with the Hurler syndrome is easily extractible from the tissue without prior treatment with proteolytic enzyme. In addiiton, amino acid-poor heparan sulfate has been demonstrated in such livers [25]. This kind of evidence, together with the demonstration that fibroblasts cultured from patients with the Hurler syndrome produce increased amounts of mucopolysaccharide [26,27], supports the hypothesis that failure to produce a normal protein-polysaccharide complex results in failure to inhibit further mucopolysaccharide production, which is both stored in the tissues and excreted in the urine.

At the present time the protein moieties have been inadequately characterized. It is not known whether the protein linked to each tissue mucopolysaccharide is a specific protein or whether the same protein is involved in the linkage with all of these mucopolysaccharides, or, indeed, whether there may not be considerable heterogeneity of the protein. The biochemical syndromes described here could thus result from differing abnormalities in a single protein or the same abnormality in different proteins. Clearly, the answer awaits analysis of tissue, rather than urine.

51

Acknowledgment: Dr. Victor A. McKusick provided twenty-three of the forty-six urine specimens which were studied. Without this cooperation, as well as Dr. McKusick's advice, this study could not have been made. In addition, I am grateful to the following physicians for providing most of the remaining urine specimens: George Ellis (Brooklyn), Barry Fisher (Cleveland), Arnold Gold (New York), W. B. Hanley (Liverpool), Frederic Kenny (Pittsburgh), John Mann (Eglin Air Force Base, Florida), Martin Moran (El Paso), John F. Murray (Los Angeles), Joseph Poindexter (New York), Charles Scott (Baltimore), Vivian Shih (Boston), Juan Sotos (Columbus) and Bruno Volk (Brooklyn). Miss Thelma Atkinson performed many of the analytic procedures.

REFERENCES

1. HUNTER, C. A rare disease in two brothers. *Proc. Roy. Soc. Med.*, 10: 104, 1917.
2. BRANTE, G. Gargoylism: a mucopolysaccharidosis. *Scandinav. J. Clin. & Lab. Invest.*, 4: 43, 1952.
3. DORFMAN, A. and LORINCZ, A. E. Occurrence of urinary acid mucopolysaccharides in the Hurler syndrome. *Proc. Nat. Acad. Sc.*, 43: 443, 1957.
4. MEYER, K., GRUMBACH, M. M., LINKER, A. and HOFFMAN, P. Excretion of sulfated mucopolysaccharides in gargoylism (Hurler's syndrome). *Proc. Soc. Exper. Biol. & Med.*, 115: 394, 1964.
5. TERRY, K. and LINKER, A. Distinction among four forms of Hurler's syndrome. *Proc. Soc. Exper. Biol. & Med.*, 115: 394, 1964.
6. McKUSICK, V. A., KAPLAN, D., WISE, D., HANLEY, W. B., SUDDARTH, S. B., SEVICK, M. E. and MAUMANEE, A. E. The genetic mucopolysaccharidoses. *Medicine*, 44: 445, 1965.
7. KAPLAN, D., McKUSICK, V. A., TREBACH, S. and LAZARUS, R. Keratosulfate-chondroitin sulfate peptide from normal urine and from urine of patients with the Morquio syndrome (mucopolysaccharidosis IV). *J. Lab. & Clin. Med.*, 71: 48, 1968.
8. DISCHE, Z. A new specific color reaction of hexuronic acids. *J. Biol. Chem.*, 167: 189, 1947.
9. BROWN, A. H. Determination of pentose in the presence of large quantities of glucose. *Arch. Biochem.*, 24: 269, 1946.
10. LOEWUS, F. A. Improvement in anthrone method for determination of carbohydrates. *Anal. Chem.*, 24: 219, 1952.
11. TREVELYAN, W. E., PROCTER, D. P. and HARRISON, J. S. Detection of sugars on paper chromatograms. *Nature*, 164: 444, 1950.
12. CIFONELLI, J. A., LUDOWIEG, J. and DORFMAN, A. Chemistry of chondroitinsulfuric acid B (β-heparin). *Fed. Proc.*, 16: 165, 1957.
13. MEYER, K. The biological significance of hyaluronic acid and hyaluronidase. *Physiol. Rev.*, 27: 335, 1947.
14. SENO, N., MEYER, K., ANDERSON, B. and HOFFMAN, P. Variations in keratosulfate. *J. Biol. Chem.*, 240: 1005, 1965.
15. TANAKA, Y. and GORE, I. Cellulose column chromatography for the fractionation and isolation of acid mucopolysaccharides. *J. Chromat.*, 23: 254, 1966.
16. SCHMIDT, M. Fractionation of acid mucopolysaccharides on DEAE Sephedex anion exchanger. *Biochim. et biophys. acta*, 63: 346, 1962.
17. RINGERTZ, N. R. and REICHARD, P. Chromatography on ECTEOLA of sulphate containing mucopolysaccharides and nucleotides. *Acta chem. scandinav.*, 13: 1467, 1959.
18. CIFONELLI, J. A., LUDOWIEG, J. and DORFMAN, A. Chemistry of β-heparin (chondroitinsulfuric acid-B). *J. Biol. Chem.*, 233: 541, 1958.
19. LINKER, A. and TERRY, K. D. Urinary acid mucopolysaccharides in normal man and in Hurler's syndrome. *Proc. Soc. Exper. Biol. & Med.*, 113: 743, 1963.
20. DIFERRANTE, N. and RICH, C. The mucopolysaccharides of normal human urine. *Clin. chim. acta*, 1: 519, 1956.
21. SANFILLIPO, S. J., PODOSIN, R., LANGER, L. O. and GOOD, R. Mental retardation associated with acid mucopolysacchariduria (heparitin sulfate type). *J. Pediat.*, 63: 837, 1963.
22. MAROTEAUX, P., LEVEQUE, B., MARIE, J. and LAMY, M. Une nouvelle dysostose avec élimination urinaire de chondroitin sulfate B. *Presse méd.* 71: 1949, 1963.
23. TELLER, W. M., ROSEVEAR, J. W. and BURKE, E. C. Identification of heterozygous carriers of gargoylism. *Proc. Soc. Exper. Biol. & Med.* 108: 276, 1961.
24. DORFMAN, A. Metabolism of acid mucopolysaccharides. *Biophys. J.*, 4 (supp.): 155, 1965.
25. KNECHT, J. and DORFMAN, A. Structure of heparitin sulfate in tissues of the Hurler syndrome. *Biochem. & Biophys. Res. Commum.* 21: 509, 1965.
26. MATALON, R. and DORFMAN, A. Hurler's syndrome: biosynthesis of acid mucopolysaccharides in tissue culture. *Proc. Nat. Acad. Sc.*, 56: 1310, 1966.
27. DANES, B. S. and BEARN, A. G. Hurler's syndrome. Effect of retinol (vitamin A alcohol) on cellular mucopolysaccharides in cultured human skin fibroblasts. *J. Exper. Med.*, 124: 1131, 1966.

The Defect in the Hurler and Scheie Syndromes: Deficiency of α-L-Iduronidase

GIDEON BACH, ROBERT FRIEDMAN,
BERNARD WEISSMANN, AND ELIZABETH F. NEUFELD

The Hurler syndrome (mucropolysaccharidosis I) is the most striking and best known of the inborn errors of mucopolysaccharide metabolism. Lysosomal deposits of mucopolysaccharide, found in nearly all cells, are no doubt responsible for the severe clinical manifestations that include skeletal deformities, hepatosplenomegaly, cloudy corneas, stunting of physical and mental growth, and cardiovascular pathology (1, 2). The mucopolysaccharides stored in the lysosomes and excreted in the urine are fragments of dermatan sulfate and heparan sulfate (2).

Fibroblasts cultured from the skin of Hurler patients likewise accumulate excessive mucopolysaccharide (3–5) because of the deficiency of a specific protein required for degradation (6). When this protein (designated "Hurler corrective factor") is supplied exogenously, mucopolysaccharide catabolism of Hurler fibroblasts is normalized.

Hurler corrective factor, purified 1000-fold from normal human urine, has no effect on the mucopolysaccharide metabolism of fibroblasts cultured from normal individuals, nor from patients with several other mucopolysaccharidoses, namely, the Hunter, Sanfilippo, and Maroteaux–Lamy syndromes (7). However, cells from individuals affected with the Scheie syndrome (mucopolysaccharidosis V) and from

53

some individuals with a phenotype intermediate between Hurler and Scheie, are likewise deficient in, and correctible by, the Hurler factor (7–9).

Barton and Neufeld (7) reported that the Hurler factor assisted Hurler and Scheie cells in degrading intracellular mucopolysaccharide (primarily dermatan sulfate), but was distinct from the common lysosomal hydrolases such as β-D-galactosidase or β-D-glucuronidase. The recent chemical synthesis of phenyl α-L-iduronide has enabled us to test the factor for α-L-iduronidase activity. α-L-Iduronidase (α-L-iduronide iduronohydrolase) activity has been detected in homogenates of human liver and cultured skin fibroblasts (10), and a preliminary characterization has been presented for the enzyme extracted from rat-liver lysosomes (11). A deficit of α-L-iduronidase in cells from individuals with the Hurler syndrome has been reported by Matalon et al. (10).

We now present evidence for the identity of Hurler corrective factor and α-L-iduronidase. The Hurler and Scheie syndromes, previously shown due to a deficiency of Hurler corrective factor, may therefore be classified as α-L-iduronidase deficiency diseases.

MATERIALS AND METHODS

Methods for culture of skin fibroblasts, as well as for the preparation and assay of Hurler corrective factor (7), and for the preparation of phenyl α- and β-L-iduronides (10a), have been described elsewhere. Purified Hurler factor had been stored at 4° in 80% ammonium sulfate; immediately before use, bovine-serum albumin was added to a final concentration of 1 mg/ml, and the mixture was exhaustively dialyzed against 0.01 M sodium phosphate buffer (pH 6.0)–0.9% NaCl.

Cell-free extracts of fibroblasts were prepared from cells grown to confluence in a 250-ml Falcon flask. Cells were detached from the plate by trypsinization, centrifuged, rinsed twice with 5 ml of 0.9% NaCl, suspended in 0.25 ml of 0.9% NaCl, and subjected to three cycles of freezing and thawing. The resultant suspension was used for enzyme assay after protein determination (12). Acetone powders were prepared from cells grown in 1410-cm² Bellco roller bottles for at least 1 month, to ensure confluence, as will be described elsewhere, and stored at -18° (Hall, Cantz, and Neufeld, in preparation). The powders were extracted at 0° immediately before use with 0.9% NaCl (0.1 ml/mg powder) and centrifuged at 10,000 $\times$ g. The supernatant fluid was used for enzyme assay after protein determination.

α-L-Iduronidase was assayed by a modification of the method of Weissmann and Santiago (11). The conditions selected—pH, time, substrate, and salt concentrations—are based on data obtained for the liver enzyme (11); because of the limited amount of substrate available, no attempt was made to optimize conditions for the urinary or fibroblast preparations. 50 μl of extract in 0.9% NaCl or Hurler corrective factor in 0.9% NaCl buffered with 0.01 M sodium phosphate (pH 6.0) were incubated with 40 μl of 0.01 M phenyl α-L-iduronide and 250 μl of 0.1 M sodium formate buffer at pH 3.5 (when unbuffered extracts were used) or at pH 3.2 (when Hurler corrective factor in buffered saline was to be tested). The formate buffers contained 0.2 M NaCl and 0.04% NaN_3. After 17 hr at ambient temperature (24°), the reaction was stopped with 1.0 ml of Folin—Ciocalteu phenol reagent (Fisher Scientific Co., diluted before use with two volumes of water) and precipitated protein was removed by centrifugation. 1 ml of the supernatant fluid was withdrawn and made alkaline with 1.5 ml of 12% Na_2CO_3; the color was developed for 20 min at 37°. Release of 0.1 μmol of phenol by the enzyme results in an absorbance of 0.60 at 660 nm.

Gas chromatographic analysis of uronic acids was performed by the procedure of Eisenberg (13), which involves reduction to aldonic acids followed by the formation of a butaneboronate derivative.

RESULTS AND DISCUSSION

α-L-Iduronidase activity of purified Hurler corrective factor

Purification of urinary Hurler factor (7) involved ammonium sulfate precipitation, gel filtration on Sephadex G-200, and chromatography on carboxymethylcellulose and, finally, on hydroxyapatite. In the last step, there occurred a resolution of factor activity into two discrete peaks, the most active fractions of which were purified 1000-fold over the starting material.

Selected fractions from the hydroxyapatite separation previously described, as well as those from a repetition of the purification procedure, were simultaneously tested for α-L-iduronidase and retested for activity of Hurler corrective factor. In both cases, two isozyme peaks of α-L-iduronidase activity were found, matching precisely the two peaks of "isofactors" in elution position (Fig. 1).

The ratio of α-L-iduronidase activity to corrective factor activity in the first peak was nearly twice that in the second peak. Presumably, some structural difference between the two isozymes may be the cause of more efficient entry of the second isozyme into Hurler cells, which in turn would result in a better correction. A freshly prepared ammonium sulfate concentrate of urinary proteins [step 1 of the purification (7)], tested at the same time, had a ratio of enzymatic to corrective

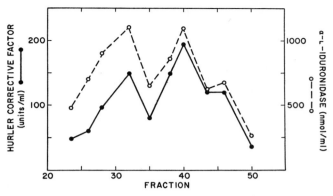

FIG. 1. Correspondence of activities of Hurler corrective factor and α-L-iduronidase in fractions eluted from hydroxyapatite (7). The α-L-iduronidase activity was measured as nmol of phenol liberated in the standard assay, and is expressed on the basis of volume of column fraction used. Activity of Hurler corrective factor is expressed on the same basis.

factor activity similar to that of the second peak. The nature of the difference between the isozymes clearly requires further study.

The second product of hydrolysis of phenyl α-L-iduronide was verified to be iduronic acid by gas–liquid chromatography of the butane boronate derivative of idonic acid. Phenyl β-L-iduronide was not hydrolyzed by Hurler corrective factor. Purified Hunter corrective factor (13a) had no α-L-iduronidase activity, nor did it affect the α-L-iduronidase activity of Hurler corrective factor when mixed with it.

Absence of intracellular α-L-iduronidase activity in fibroblasts of patients with Hurler and Scheie Syndromes

Extracts prepared from acetone powders of fibroblasts, or from freshly harvested fibroblasts, were examined for α-L-iduronidase activity. As summarized in Table 1, cells from patients with the Hunter, Sanfilippo, Maroteaux–Lamy, or Morquio syndromes (1), or from patients with atypical mucopolysaccharidoses, such as β-glucuronidase deficiency (14) and "gal +" mucopolysaccharidosis (15, 16), have normal α-L-iduronidase activity. Extracts devoid of α-L-iduronidase activity were obtained from cells of four Hurler patients, one Scheie patient, and one patient reported to have a novel mucopolysaccharidosis (17), but probably fitting the clinical picture of a patient who might have one Hurler and one Scheie gene (a genetic compound, ref. 9). These six lines of

TABLE 1. *α-L-Iduronidase activity in cell-free extracts of cultured fibroblasts*

Extract	Fibroblasts	Enzyme activity, nmol phenol liberated per 17 hr per mg of protein*
Acetone powder		
	Hurler (J.F.)	0
	Normal	550
	Normal	1000
	Hunter	920
	Sanfilippo A	680
	Sanfilippo B	840
	Maroteaux-Lamy	660
	Morquio	1100
	β-Glucuronidase deficiency	830
	"Gal +"	430
	I-cell	90
Frozen-thawed		
	Hurler (M.B.)	17
	Hurler (C.P.)	9
	Hurler (M.W.)	0
	Scheie (M.Mc.)	11
	Hurler/Scheie (R.S.)	0
	Normal	800
	Hunter	1600

* Values corrected for enzyme blank. Apparent activity of 20 nmol of phenol liberated in the assay per mg of protein is within experimental error of zero activity.

fibroblasts had been previously found deficient in Hurler corrective factor. In addition, α-L-iduronidase activity was low (though detectable) in fibroblasts from a patient with I-cell disease—an unusual genetic disorder characterized by the deficiency of several lysosomal enzymes in fibroblasts (18–20), as well as of Hurler and Hunter corrective factors in fibroblast secretions (21). A profound deficiency of α-L-iduronidase in fibroblasts of Hurler and I-cell patients, as well as in liver and urine of Hurler patients, has also been reported by Matalon and Dorfman (22).

Absence of α-L-iduronidase is not a function of storage time of acetone powders, nor of time between transplantation and harvest of fibroblasts, since the iduronidase-positive and

TABLE 2. *Relationship of correction to uptake of*
α-L-iduronidase

Applied in medium		Recovered in cells		Correction* (% of maximum)
Corrective factor (units/ plate)	Iduronidase (μunits†/ plate)	Iduronidase (μunits†/ plate)	Uptake of iduronidase‡	
10	175	65	0.37	90
30	525	84	0.16·	97
100	1750	160	0.09	99

* Theoretical value, calculated from the number of corrective factor units applied, as described in (7).

† 1 μunit corresponds to the release of 1 nmol of phenol in 1000 min.

‡ Ratio of iduronidase activity recovered in cells to that applied in medium.

iduronidase-negative cultures were matched with respect to these variables. Mixing the acetone-powder extract of cells of J.F. with that of normal cells gave the calculated average activity; thus, absence of α-L-iduronidase activity in Hurler cells cannot be attributed to the presence of a soluble inhibitor.

α-L-Iduronidase is the only lysosomal enzyme known to be deficient in fibroblasts from patients with the Hurler syndrome. The acetone powder of J.F. cells had normal levels of β-D-galactosidase, α-D-mannosidase, α-L-fucosidase, and arylsulfatase A activities, and elevated β-N-acetyl-D-glucosaminidase, β-N-acetyl-D-galactosaminidase, and β-D-glucuronidase activities.

It is clear that deficiency of α-L-iduronidase activity can be used for the diagnosis of the Hurler and Scheie syndromes. The enzymatic test is as specific as the bioassay for Hurler corrective factor, and is simpler to perform. The sensitivity of the two tests is similar, requiring about 1–2 mg of cell protein (about 2–4 × 10⁶ cells). The α-L-iduronidase assay will therefore not materially reduce the time (5 weeks or even longer) now required for antenatal diagnosis of the Hurler syndrome by assay of the Hurler corrective factor in cultured amniotic fluid cells (23).

Uptake of α-L-iduronidase by Hurler cells
For determination of the relationship between uptake of α-L-iduronidase and correction an unpurified concentrate of urinary proteins, of measured enzymatic and corrective activity, was applied to cells of a Hurler patient (M.W.) under

conditions standardized for assay of corrective factor (7). After 48 hr, cells were harvested and intracellular α-L-iduronidase activity was measured (Table 2).

Several points emerge from the results of this experiment. First, maximal correction is not a function of saturation of some transport system for the α-L-iduronidase, since the uptake of the enzyme increases substantially beyond the point of 90% correction. As previously suggested (7), maximal correction is probably reached when the concentration of the product of the added α-L-iduronidase (i.e., dermatan sulfate chains from which the terminal iduronic acid has been removed) becomes saturating for subsequent enzymes in the catabolic chain.

Second, the uptake of α-L-iduronidase from the medium is remarkably efficient, approaching 40% at the lowest level used. This should be compared to a measured uptake of less than 1% for ^{125}I-labeled albumin under similar conditions. The uptake of α-L-iduronidase is clearly attributable to a selective mechanism, rather than to nonspecific pinocytosis.

Finally, the amount of intracellular α-L-iduronidase required to give 90% or higher correction is but a fraction of the normal level of that enzyme (compare with Table 1). Normal cells are apparently supplied with a large excess of α-L-iduronidase, a finding consistent with the normal phenotype of Hurler heterozygotes. One might predict, accordingly, that therapeutic attempts at activation or replacement of the deficient enzyme would be successful if the Hurler patient were provided with only a low level of α-L-iduronidase activity. Indeed, the modest requirement of cells for α-L-iduronidase may explain, in part, the surprising effects of infusing Hurler patients with normal plasma, which has very little activity of Hurler factor (24).

We thank Dr. Frank Eisenberg for the gas chromatographic analyses. This work was supported in part by Grant AM 02479 from the National Institutes of Health.

1. McKusick, V. A. (1966) in *Heritable Disorders of Connective Tissue* (C. V. Mosby, St. Louis), pp. 325–399.
2. Dorfman, A. & Matalon, R. (1972) in *The Metabolic Basis of Inherited Disease*, eds. Stanbury, J. B., Wyngaarden, J. B. & Fredrickson, D. S. (McGraw Hill, New York), pp. 1218–1272.
3. Danes, B. S. & Bearn, A. G. (1966) *J. Exp. Med.* **123**, 1–16.
4. Matalon, R. & Dorfman, A. (1966) *Proc. Nat. Acad. Sci. USA* **56**, 1310–1316.
5. Fratantoni, J. C., Hall, C. W. & Neufeld, E. F. (1968) *Proc. Nat. Acad. Sci. USA* **60**, 699–706.
6. Fratantoni, J. C., Hall, C. W. & Neufeld, E. F. (1969) *Proc. Nat. Acad. Sci. USA* **64**, 360–366.
7. Barton, R. W. & Neufeld, E. F. (1971) *J. Biol. Chem.* **246**, 7773–7779.

8. Wiesmann, U. & Neufeld, E. F. (1970) *Science* **169**, 72–74.
9. McKusick, V. A., Howell, R. R., Hussels, I. E., Neufeld, E. F. & Stevenson, R. E. (1972) *Lancet* 1, 993–996.
10. Matalon, R., Cifonelli, J. A. & Dorfman, A. (1971) *Biochem. Biophys. Res. Commun.* **42**, 340–344.
10*a*. Friedman, R. & Weissmann, B. (1972) *Carbohyd. Res.*, in press.
11. Weissmann, B. & Santiago, R. (1972) *Biochem. Biophys. Res. Commun.* **46**, 1430–1433.
12. Lowry, O. H., Rosebrough, N. J., Farr, A. L. & Randall, R. J. (1951) *J. Biol. Chem.* **193**, 265–275.
13. Eisenberg, F., Jr. (1971) *Carbohyd. Res.* **19**, 135–138.
13*a*. Cantz, M., Chrambach, A., Bach, G. & Neufeld, E. F. (1972) *J. Biol. Chem.*, in press.
14. Quinton, B. A., Sly, W. S., McAlister, W. H., Rimoin, D. L., Hall, C. W. & Neufeld, E. F. (1971) *Abstr. Pediatr. Meetings, Atlantic City*, p. 198.
15. v. Hoof, F. & Hers, H. G. (1968) *Eur. J. Biochem.* **7**, 34–44.
16. Loeb, H., Tondeur, M., Toppet, A. & Cremer, N. (1969) *Acta Paediat. Scand.* **58**, 220–228.
17. Horton, W. A. & Schimke, R. N. (1970) *J. Pediat.* **77**, 252–258.
18. Lightbody, J., Wiesmann, U., Hadorn, B. & Herschkowitz, N. (1971) *Lancet* I, 451.
19. Leroy, J. G., Spranger, J. W., Feingold, M., Optiz, J. M. & Crocker, A. C. (1971) *J. Pediat.* **79**, 360–365.
20. Tondeur, M., Vamos-Hurwitz, E., Mockel-Pohl, S., Dereume, J. P., Cremer, N. & Loeb, H. (1971) *J. Pediat.* **79**, 366–378.
21. Neufeld, E. F. & Cantz, M. (1971) *Ann. N.Y. Acad. Sci.* **179**, 580–587.
22. Matalon, R. & Dorfman, A. (1972) *Biochem. Biophys. Res. Commun.* **47**, 959–964.
23. Neufeld, E. F. (1972) in *Antenatal Diagnosis*, ed. Dorfman, A. (University of Chicago Press, Chicago), pp. 217–228.
24. diFerrante, N., Nichols, B. L., Donnelly, P. V., Neri, G., Hrgovcic, R. & Berglund, R. K. (1971) *Proc. Nat. Acad. Sci. USA* **68**, 303–307.

Carbohydrate Metabolism Disorders

Fabry's Disease: Evidence for a Physically Altered α-Galactosidase

Mae Wan Ho, Steven Beutler, Linda Tennant, and John S. O'Brien

INTRODUCTION

Fabry's disease is an X-linked metabolic disorder characterized by the progressive accumulation of ceramide trihexoside in tissues and body fluids [1, 2]. The galactosyl hydrolase (ceramide trihexosidase) responsible for the breakdown of this glycosphingolipid is deficient in hemizygous males afflicted with the disease [3]. Following the demonstration of α-galactosidase deficiency in Fabry's disease [4], the structure of ceramide trihexoside was shown to include an α-anomeric linkage of the terminal galactosyl residue [5]. The α-galactosidase activity is deficient in cultured skin fibroblasts from patients with Fabry's disease. Heterozygous females have two distinct clonal populations, one α-galactositlase deficient, the other not, consistent with Lyonization of the X-linked locus [6].

The question is whether the α-galactosidase deficiency in Fabry's disease represents a structural gene mutation or a mutation of a regulatory gene on the X chromosome. The latter possibility has recently been entertained by Beutler and Kuhl [7]. We set out to explore the problem by a careful study of the physical properties of α-galactosidase in normal subjects and in patients with Fabry's disease.

MATERIALS AND METHODS

Skin fibroblasts were cultured from skin biopsies obtained from patients with Fabry's disease in two kindreds and from normal subjects as previously described [8].

Liver obtained at autopsy from a patient with Fabry's disease was stored frozen prior to analysis and was kindly supplied by Dr. Howard Sloan. Control livers were obtained at autopsy from subjects who did not have Fabry's disease; the livers were stored frozen for 3 years.

The α-galactosidase activity was assayed using 4-methylumbelliferyl-α-D-galactopyranoside (Koch Light, England) as substrate. A 10-μl aliquot of homogenate or enzyme solution was incubated for 30 min and 60 min with 50 μl of 0.02 M citrate phosphate buffer (pH 4.5) containing 0.5 μmole of substrate. Other acid glycosidase activities were assayed as described [8].

The Michaelis constant (K_m) was obtained graphically by the Lineweaver-Burke

This work was supported by a fellowship from the National Genetics Foundation to M. W. Ho; grants from the National Cystic Fibrosis Foundation and the National Genetics Foundation; and grant NB 08682 from the National Institutes of Health.

method. Each experiment was carried out in triplicate and repeated two to three times to obtain a mean value.

Isoelectricfocusing was performed as recommended by the manufacturer (LKB Instruments, Stockholm) using 1% ampholyte (pH 3–10) in a gradient of 0%–50% glycerol. The temperature was maintained at 5° C with a circulating water bath (Brinkmann). Electrofocusing was allowed to proceed for 60 hr at a starting voltage of 300 v. The voltage at the end of focusing was 380 v. The column was then allowed to drain and the effluent collected in fractions of 1–1.5 ml. The pH in each fraction was measured at the temperature of electrofocusing with a Beckman pH meter.

Gel filtration was performed as described [9].

Starch gel electrophoresis was performed as described elsewhere [10].

Neuraminidase (*Clostridium perfringens*, Sigma Type VI) was added to samples at a concentration of 1 mg milliliter. The pH was adjusted to 5.0 with citrate-phosphate buffer (5 mM in terms of phosphate, final concentration). Incubation was carried out at 37° C for various time periods.

RESULTS AND DISCUSSION

The pH Activity and K_m

The pH activity curve of α-galactosidase in skin fibroblasts and in liver was similar; optimal activity was found in the region of pH 4.5. No difference in pH optima was evident when activity in skin fibroblasts from controls, heterozygotes, and hemizygotes was compared.

The K_m for α-galactosidase in controls was 4×10^{-3} M, and was the same in the skin fibroblasts and in liver. Again, the same K_m was found for the enzyme in skin fibroblasts from controls, heterozygotes, and hemizygotes.

Specific Activities

The specific activities of α-galactosidase and other glycosidases in skin fibroblasts are presented in table 1. The activity of α-galactosidase in hemizygotes ranged from 30% to 39% of the control mean. This is considerably higher than

TABLE 1

ACID GLYCOSIDASE ACTIVITIES IN SKIN FIBROBLASTS

	α-Galacto-sidase	β-Galacto-sidase	β-Gluco-sidase	β-Glucosam-inidase
Hemizygotes:				
1	21.40	588.9	27.09	4,759
2	25.90	747.2	65.12	4,406
3	19.97	424.2	57.20	2,802
Presumed heterozygotes:				
1	47.70	565.2	45.20	4,288
2	41.96	417.8	40.15	5,482
3	34.30	427.8	...	3,434
4	26.50	346.4	...	2,537
Controls:				
N	7	29	14	27
Mean $\pm$ SD	66.0 $\pm$ 12	578 $\pm$ 138	40.7 $\pm$ 11.2	4,715 $\pm$ 974
Range	57–88	304–949	25.1–56.7	2,427–6,431

NOTE.—Enzyme activities expressed as nmole substrate cleaved per milligram protein per hour.

levels previously reported in skin fibroblasts from affected patients [6] and may reflect different conditions of tissue culture and enzyme assay. Obligate heterozygotes (mothers and daughters of patients) all had intermediate levels of enzyme activity, although the spread of values varied widely between 40% and 72% of the control mean.

In the frozen liver specimen from a patient with Fabry's disease, α-galactosidase activity was reduced to 17.5% of the control mean (7.27 nmole/milligram protein per hour compared with a control mean of 41.6 ± 15.6). All other glycosidase activities tested were within the range of controls.

Thermostability

Rates of thermal inactivation of α-galactosidase at 50° C in control skin fibroblasts and control livers were similar (fig. 1). This fact, coupled with the identical

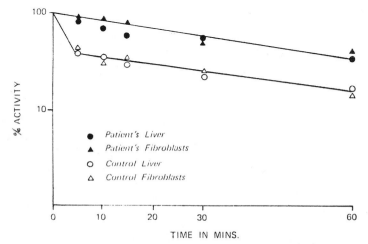

Fig. 1.—Heat inactivation of α-galactosidase in homogenates of skin fibroblasts and livers. Samples (10 μl containing 10–30 μg protein) were maintained at 50° C in small test tubes sealed with parafilm in 5 mM sodium phosphate buffer (pH 7.0) for various time periods. Residual activity was assayed at 37° C as described in the Materials and Methods section.

K_m and pH curves, indicates that skin fibroblast and liver α-galactosidase(s) are probably the same. An inflection of the thermal inactivation curves at approximately 5 min suggested the presence of more than one form of α-galactosidase. This was verified after electrofocusing (see below).

Thermal inactivation of α-galactosidase from hemizygotes indicated a relatively more stable α-galactosidase which was slowly inactivated (fig. 1). The kinetics of inactivation gave a single slope, suggesting that a single component was present. This also was verified on electrofocusing. Thermal inactivation of α-galactosidase in cultured skin fibroblasts from heterozygotes gave kinetics which were virtually indistinguishable from controls. One interpretation of these data is that there is

64

an absence of a thermolabile α-galactosidase(s) in Fabry's disease, with selective preservation of a thermostable α-galactosidase.

Separation Techniques

In order to more clearly define the nature of the multiple forms of α-galactosidase, they were separated from liver as follows:

Starch gel electrophoresis. Starch gel electrophoresis was performed on the control and the patient's liver supernatants (100,000 g). Two main bands of α-galactosidase activity (A, B) were seen in control livers, migrating close to one another toward the anode. The α-galactosidase in the patient's liver migrated as a single narrow band in a position similar to that of the slower-moving band (B) in the control livers (fig. 2).

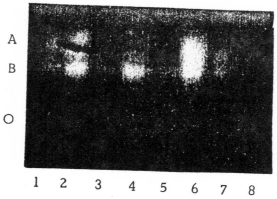

Fig. 2.—Starch gel electrophoresis of α-galactosidase in liver. Lanes *1, 2, 4, 6, 8*—control liver samples; lanes *3, 5*—liver from patient. A homogenate (14% w/v) of the livers was centrifuged at 100,000 g to obtain a clear supernatant which was applied to the gel.

Isoelectricfocusing. Electrofocusing gave a total of seven peaks of α-galactosidase activity in the control livers (fig. 3a) with corresponding isoelectric pHs of 6.8, 6.4, 4.6, 4.34, 3.8, 3.74, and 3.6. The α-glactosidase activity in the patient's liver appeared as a single peak isoelectric at pH 4.3 (fig. 3b). The β-galactosidase and N-acetyl-β-glucosaminidase activities fractionated identically in both the control and the patient's liver.

A comparison of the properties of the different peaks of α-galactosidase activities is summarized in table 2. On starch gel electrophoresis, peak I and peak II α-galactosidases appear as very faint bands at the origin. Their thermal inactivation curves were intermediate between those of the thermolabile components (peaks III, V, VI, VII) and the thermostable component (peak VI; fig. 4). Their pH optimum of 4.35 is also intermediate between that of the labile components (pH 4.1–4.35) and the stable component (pH 4.6). Peaks I and II could represent molecular aggregates of enzymes in the five major peaks (III–VII).

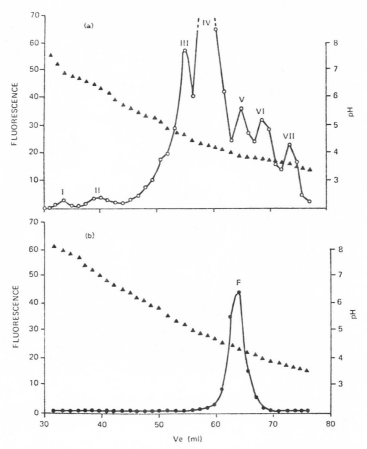

Fig. 3.—Isoelectricfocusing of α-galactosidase. (a), Control liver supernatant. (b), Patient's liver supernatant. From each fraction, 10 μl was assayed for α-galactosidase activity as described in the Materials and Methods section.

Peak III and peak IV α-galactosidases migrate as band B on starch gel electrophoresis, whereas peak V, VI, and VII α-galactosidases migrate as band A. Thus, the electrophoretic migration of the major α-galactosidases in control liver is predictable from their isoelectric points if it is assumed that all possess the same molecular weights.

Examination of the thermal inactivation curves of α-galactosidases from control liver at 50° C (fig. 4) demonstrates that one component is relatively thermostable (peak IV); this component accounts for about 50% of the total α-galactosidase activity present. The other components (peaks III, V, VI, VII) are thermolabile. All components had the same K_m value of 4×10^{-3} M, identical with that found using the total liver homogenate.

TABLE 2

PROPERTIES OF α-GALACTOSIDASE PEAKS FROM ELECTROFOCUSING

	CONTROL							FABRY'S (F)
	I	II	III	IV	V	VI	VII	
Isoelectric pH	6.8	6.4	4.6	4.34	3.8	3.74	3.6	4.3
pH optimum	4.35	4.35	4.35	4.6	4.1	4.1	4.1	4.6
Specific activity*	32.6	33.8	293.8	1,645	111.3	90	61.9	386.6
Thermostability (%)†	4.5	6	1.7	72	9	10	1.5	70
Electrophoretic migration ..	0	0	B	B	A	A	A	B

NOTE.—$K_m = 4 \times 10^{-3}$ M for all entries.

* nmole per milligram protein per hour.

† Percentage activity remaining after 15 min at 50° C, pH 7.0.

Peak F, the single peak of α-galactosidase activity in the liver of the patient with Fabry's disease, was similar to peak IV with respect to isoelectric pH, pH optimum, K_m, electrophoretic migration, and relative thermostability.

Our data thus far demonstrate the selective loss of multiple thermolabile α-galactosidases in the tissues of patients with Fabry's disease. Two possibilities present themselves.

a) The thermolabile and thermostable components of α-galactosidase are genetically distinct proteins, and the mutation in Fabry's disease affects only the thermolabile components.

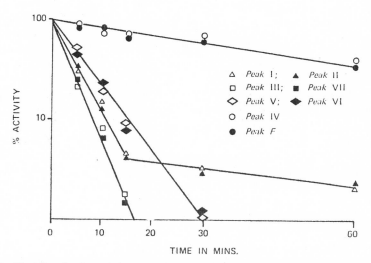

FIG. 4.—Heat inactivation of the α-galactosidase peaks isolated on isoelectricfocusing. Fractions containing the highest enzyme activity in each peak were used after dialysis against 5 mM sodium phosphate buffer (pH 7.0) overnight (other conditions as in fig. 1)

b) The thermolabile and thermostable components are modifications of the same primary polypeptide backbone. In this case, the defect could be:

   i) A mutation of the locus responsible for the modification of the primary polypeptide to form the thermolabile components.
   ii) A mutation of the locus which codes for the polypeptide backbone of the enzyme, which so changed its structure that its conversion to the thermolabile forms is impeded.
   iii) A mutation (regulatory) affecting the rate of synthesis of the polypeptide.

Differentiation among α-Galactosidases

The key question to answer next is the relationship among the different forms of α-galactosidase, especially the thermolabile and the thermostable forms.

Gel filtration. Gel filtration gave a single peak of α-galactosidase activity corresponding to a molecular weight of about 90,000 in both control and the patient's liver supernatant. This indicates that all species of the enzyme have a single molecular weight.

Neuraminidase treatment. The multiple forms of α-galactosidase apparent after electrofocusing and to a lesser degree after starch gel electrophoresis may indicate the progressive addition of some negatively charged small molecules such as N-acetyl-neuraminic acid (NANA) to the polypeptide. This possibility seemed attractive since others have reported conversions of acid hydrolases from one form to another by the removal of neuraminic acid residues using neuraminidase [11, 12].

Neuraminidase treatment of control liver supernatants resulted in the rapid conversion of all electrophoretically fast-moving forms of α-galactosidase to a single slow-moving form (fig. 5). Attempts to observe intermediate stages of conversion were not successful, since under the present conditions, conversion was essentially completed within 15 min of incubation at 37° C. No spontaneous conversion of enzymic forms occurred in the absence of neuraminidase at 0° C or 37° C.

The α-galactosidase activity in the patient's liver supernatant was not converted to any slower-moving form on starch gel electrophoresis. Conversion of the fast-moving α-galactosidase to the slow-moving form was observed in a 1:1 mixture of the control and the patient's liver supernatants.

Neuraminidase treatment resulted in no loss of total enzyme activity in either the control or the patient's liver supernatant. Quantitative recovery of α-galactosidase activity was obtained after neuraminidase treatment. The possibility that the faster-moving forms of α-galactosidase were inactivated by the neuraminidase treatment was ruled out. Each fast-moving α-galactosidase was converted to the slow-moving form presumably by the reduction of negative charges occasioned on the removal of NANA residues.

Isoelectricfocusing after neuraminidase treatment. After neuraminidase treatment, both the control and the patient's liver supernatants gave a single peak of α-galactosidase activity which was isoelectric at *p*H 4.6—identical with the original peak III in control liver.

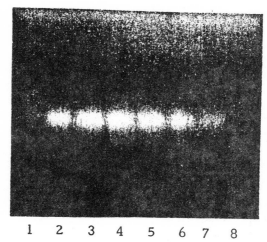

FIG. 5.—Starch gel electrophoresis of α-galactosidase treated with neuraminidase. Lane *1*, sample without neuraminidase and not incubated. Lanes *2, 3*, samples with neuraminidase incubated for 15 min. Lanes *4–7*, samples with neuraminidase incubated for 1/2, 1, 2, and 3 hr, respectively. Lane *8*, sample without neuraminidase incubated for 2 hr.

Properties of the α-galactosidase peaks after neuraminidase treatment. The properties of the neuraminidase-treated single α-galactosidases from the control (peak Cn) and the patient's liver (peak Fn) were compared with one another and with peaks III and IV (α-galactosidase) from control liver and peak F (α-galactosidase) from the patient's liver (table 3). The isoelectric pH, K_m, and pH optima

TABLE 3

PROPERTIES OF LIVER α-GALACTOSIDASE PEAKS ISOLATED BY ELECTROFOCUSING

	UNTREATED			NEURAMINIDASE TREATED	
	III	IV	Fabry's (F)	Control (Cn)	Fabry's (Fn)
Isoelectric pH	4.6	4.34	4.3	4.6	4.6
pH optimum	4.35	4.6	4.6	4.35	4.35
Thermostability (%)*	1.4	72	77	1.6	68
Electrophoretic migration ..	B	B	B	B	B

NOTE.—$K_m = 4 \times 10^{-3}$ M for all entries.
* Percentage activity remaining after 15 min at 50° C, pH 7.0.

of peaks Cn and Fn were identical with those of peak III. As stated earlier, peak F and peak IV had the same isoelectric pH and pH optima, which differed from the aforementioned peaks. However, examination of the thermal inactivation curves revealed that the activity isolated from peak Cn was thermolabile like that of peak

III in the untreated liver, but activity from peak Fn was thermostable, as was that from peak F (fig. 6).

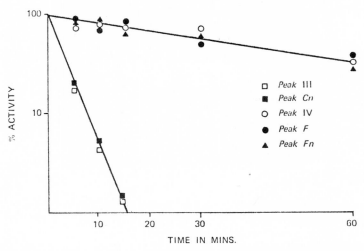

Fig. 6.—Heat inactivation of α-galactosidase peaks isolated on isoelectricfocusing of liver supernatants before and after neuraminidase treatment. Fractions containing the highest enzyme activity in each peak were used after dialysis against 5 mM sodium phosphate buffer, pH 7.0 (other conditions as in fig. 1).

The possibility was considered that a protease was a component of peak Cn, thus causing greater destruction of the normal α-galactosidase activity during heat inactivation. This was ruled out by diluting the material from peak Cn tenfold and repeating the heat inactivation: the kinetics of inactivation in the diluted sample was identical with that of the original preparation. The possibility that a soluble stabilizing substance was a part of peak Fn, protecting its activity during heat inactivation, was also considered. This was ruled out by demonstrating that an equal mixture of material from peaks Cn and Fn gave the expected intermediate thermal inactivation curve.

The evidence presented here suggests that the deficiency of α-galactosidase in Fabry's disease could be the result of a structural gene mutation of the α-galactosidase polypeptide chain. The absence of the faster-moving thermolabile forms of α-galactosidase in the patient's liver can be interpreted to mean that the mutant enzyme is so structurally altered as to become a poor acceptor of sialic acid residues. Obviously, this remains to be confirmed in vitro. The alternative hypothesis is the deficiency of a specific NANA-transferase which transfers NANA-residues to the α-galactosidase polypeptide chain to convert it to faster-moving forms. Sialyl transferases of such high specificity (for the acceptor protein) are yet unknown; moreover, such a deficiency does not account for the decrease in enzyme activity which is presumably due to a reduction in specific activity of the structurally altered enzyme.

It is, however, necessary to correlate the deficiency of ceramide trihexosidase in Fabry's disease with the mutation of α-galactosidase. The activity of the different forms of the enzyme toward the accumulating glycolipid needs to be examined. These and other experiments are in progress.

SUMMARY

Starch gel electrophoresis and isoelectricfocusing demonstrate the existence of multiple forms of α-galactosidase, active against 4-methylumbelliferyl-α-D-galactopyranoside, in normal human liver. These forms differ in isoelectric pH, pH optimum, and thermostability, but have identical Michaelis constants and molecular weights. On treatment with neuraminidase, the more acidic, rapidly migrating forms of α-galactosidase are completely converted to a single slowly migrating form with an isoelectric point of pH 4.6.

The α-galactosidase in the liver of a patient with Fabry's disease exists as a single component similar to one of the forms of α-galactosidase from control liver which is isoelectric at pH 4.3. Neuraminidase treatment completely converted the patient's liver α-galactosidase to a form similar in isoelectric pH (pH 4.6), K_m, and pH optimum to the single component in normal liver found after neuraminidase treatment. However, the neuraminidase-treated enzyme from the patient's liver was thermostable, whereas the enzyme from control liver was thermolabile.

Our evidence suggests that the α-galactosidase in Fabry's disease is a physically altered enzyme. The defect may involve a structural gene mutation resulting in an alteration in the polypeptide chain of α-galactosidase.

ACKNOWLEDGMENTS

We thank Drs. Daniel Marnell and William Nyhan for referring patients to us. Dr. Howard Sloan has kindly supplied us with fresh frozen liver tissue from a patient who died of Fabry's disease. The skin fibroblast lines used in this study were cultured by Mrs. M. Lois Veath.

REFERENCES

1. SWEELEY CC, KLIONSKY B: Fabry's disease: classification as sphingolipidosis and partial characterization of a novel glycolipid. *J Biol Chem* 238: PC 3148–3150, 1963
2. SCHIBANOFF JM, KAMOSHITA S, O'BRIEN JS: Tissue distribution of glycosphingolipids in a case of Fabry's disease. *J Lipid Res* 10:515–520, 1966
3. BRADY RO, GAL AE, BRADLEY RM, et al: Enzymatic defect in Fabry's disease: ceramidetrihexosidase deficiency. *New Eng J Med* 276:1163–1167, 1967
4. KINT JA: Fabry's disease: alpha-galactosidase deficiency. *Science* 167:1268–1269, 1970
5. HAKOMORI S-I, SIDDIQUIR B, LI Y-T, et al: Anomeric structures of globoside and ceramide trihexoside of human erythrocytes and hamster fibroblasts. *J Biol Chem* 246:2271–2277, 1971
6. ROMEO G, MIGEON BR: Genetic inactivation of the α-galactosidase locus in carriers of Fabry's disease. *Science* 170:180–181, 1971
7. BEUTLER E, KUHL W: Biochemical and electrophoretic studies of α-galactosidase in normal man, in patients with Fabry's disease, and in Equidae. *Amer J Hum Genet* 24:237–249, 1972
8. Ho MW, SECK J, SCHMIDT D, et al: Adult Gaucher's disease: kindred studies and

demonstration of a deficiency of acid β-glucosidase in cultured fibroblasts. *Amer J Hum Genet* 24:37–45, 1972

9. Ho MW, O'BRIEN JS: Gaucher's disease: deficiency of acid β-glucosidase and reconstitution of enzyme activity in vitro. *Proc Nat Acad Sci USA* 68:2810–2813, 1971

10. Ho MW, O'BRIEN JS: Differential effects of chloride ions on β-galactosidase isoenzymes: a method for separate assay. *Clin Chim Acta* 32:443–450, 1971

11. ROBINSON D, STERLING JL: N-acetyl-β-glucosaminidases in human spleen. *Biochem J* 107:321–327, 1968

12. GOLDSTONE A, KONECNY P, KOENIG H: Lysosomal hydrolases: conversion of acidic to basic forms by neuraminidase. *FEBS Letters* 13:68–72, 1971

Fabry's Disease: Differentiation between Two Forms of α-Galactosidase by Myoinositol

JOHN C. CRAWHALL
MARIANNE BANFALVI

Fabry's disease is an X-linked recessively inherited disorder, characterized by deposition of the glycolipid ceramide trihexoside in various organs of the body; depositions are frequently associated with blood vessels. It can give rise to a characteristic skin lesion, angiokeratoma, and the patients may die in middle age of a cerebral artery hemorrhage or renal failure (1). There is a specific defect of ceramide trihexosidase in the gut mucosa of these patients (2), and a defect of α-galactosidase has been detected in circulating leukocytes and cultured skin fibroblasts (3). In contrast to the findings in the latter report, we find that the deficiency of this enzyme is not complete but that residual enzyme activity is between 10 and 20 percent of that found in normal cells. There are three possible explanations for this. (i) Fabry's disease is associated with a regulatory gene defect that reduces the quantity of the normal enzyme being formed. (ii) The residual enzyme ac-

Table 1. α-Galactosidase activity and corresponding K_m values of cultured fibroblasts. Cultured cells were sonicated (Branson Sonifier), and the substrate, 4-methylumbelliferyl-α-galactoside, was dissolved in 0.1M acetate buffer (pH 5.0). The reaction mixture, consisting of 20 μl of sonicated material and 180 μl of substrate (1 μmole, 5 mM final concentration) was incubated at 37°C for 2 hours. The reaction was stopped by addition of 2.8 ml of glycine buffer (pH 10.5), and the fluorescence was measured in an Aminco Bowman spectrophotofluorimeter (exciting wavelength, 360 nm; fluorescence, 450 nm) and compared with 4-methylumbelliferone as standard; K_m values were determined for extracts of normal cells (0.5 to 5 mM substrate) and for cell extracts of patients with Fabry's disease (5 to 25 mM substrate).

Enzyme activity (nanomoles of substrate hydrolyzed per milligram of protein per hour)		K_m (mM)	
Normal	Fabry's disease	Normal	Fabry's disease
51.2 ± 18.1*	7.4	3.34	22.2
	5.9	2.89	28.6
	7.7	3.95	14.3

* Mean and standard deviation from 14 determinations carried out on eight different strains of normal cells.

73

tivity arises from a structural gene mutation modifying the structure of the normal enzyme. (iii) Two or more isoenzymes for α-galactosidase exist, the principal one of which is missing in Fabry's disease. In that case the missing enzyme might represent the true ceramide trihexosidase.

We have investigated these three possibilities by studying the reaction of the enzyme with the artificial substrate 4-methylumbelliferyl-α-galactoside and have used the techniques of determination of Michaelis constant (K_m), heat inactivation, and specific inhibition of the enzyme. Three patients with Fabry's disease were studied. One patient had typical angiokeratoma, and one had no angiokeratoma but a significant family history of Fabry's disease. This patient developed renal failure with the renal and urinary glycolipid findings characteristic of Fabry's disease. The third patient had no angiokeratoma or renal failure but did have proteinuria and the renal histology and urinary glycolipids characteristic of Fabry's disease. Details of these last two patients have been reported (4). Since myoinositol was a selective inhibitor of various plant α-galactosidases when p-nitrophenyl-α-galactoside was used as a substrate (5), we studied the effect of this inhibitor on the α-galactosidase activity of cultured skin fibroblasts from the patients with Fabry's disease and from normal control cells. The total enzyme activity of these cell strains and their corresponding K_m values are shown in Table 1.

The rate of heat inactivation of α-galactosidase in these cell strains was measured. The enzyme from the normal cell lines was rapidly inactivated at 51 °C over a period of 60 minutes. After longer periods of heating, the rate of heat inactivation was much slower and closely paralleled that found for the residual enzyme activity in the cell strains from

patients with Fabry's disease. The K_m values were again determined on the residual α-galactosidase activity present in a normal cell strain after heat inactivation, and the K_m of this residual

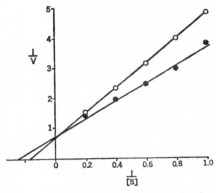

Fig. 1. Lineweaver-Burke plot showing myoinositol as a competitive inhibitor of α-galactosidase in sonicated normal skin fibroblasts. The enzyme was assayed as described in the legend to Table 1. The reaction velocity, V, is expressed as nanomoles per milligram of protein per hour. The reciprocal of this velocity has been multiplied by 10^2 to obtain the values on the vertical axis. The substrate concentration, [S], is millimolar. The concentration of the inhibitor, myoinositol, was 100 mM. The K_m calculated for the normal enzyme was 3.95 mM and that for the inhibited enzyme was 6.0 mM (●—●, α-galactosidase activity without myoinositol; ○—○, α-galactosidase activity with myoinositol).

enzyme was 19.5 mM, as compared to 4.0 mM for enzyme activity before heat treatment.

The inhibition of α-galactosidase activity in the presence of myoinositol was then studied. Myoinositol appeared to be a competitive inhibitor of the normal enzyme (Fig. 1) and was most effective at 500 mM, the highest concentration of substrate compatible with keeping the substrate in solution. In contrast, the enzyme activity present in cell extracts from patients with Fabry's disease was not inhibited by myoinositol at any inhibitor concentration; in fact it seemed to have a mild stimulatory effect on some cell strains. Experiments combining heat inactivation and myoinositol inhibition were then carried out; an example is shown in Fig. 2. Myoinositol is an inhibitor of α-galactosidase obtained from a normal cell strain, but during the period of heat inactivation, when the α-galactosidase activity is decreased, the effect of myoinositol as an inhibitor also decreases; after 60 minutes of heat inactivation no inhibition of the enzyme is observed. This could be explained by the hypothesis that all the heat-labile enzyme is destroyed, leaving the heat-stable enzyme characteristic of Fabry's disease, which is not inhibited by myoinositol. The residual enzyme activity of the normal cell extract is quantitatively similar to that found in the cell extracts from patients with Fabry's disease. Myoinositol had a mild stimulatory effect on patients' cell extracts as compared with the inhibitory effect on the normal cell extract (Fig. 2). Myoinositol had no inhibitory effect on the β-galactosidase activity in fibroblasts.

These observations are not compatible with the hypothesis of a regulator gene defect nor of a structural gene variation giving rise to an atypical enzyme. They do support the hypothesis, proposed on the basis of K_m data and electrophoretic separation of two different enzymes from leukocytes (6), that there is a separate heat-labile enzyme that is absent in the X-linked condition Fabry's disease. The present experiments demonstrate that the residual α-galactosidase enzyme found in fibroblast cells of patients with Fabry's disease is characterized by its higher K_m, its resistance to heat inactivation, and the lack of inhibition by myoinositol.

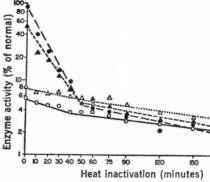

Fig. 2. Effect of heat inactivation and myoinositol on α-galactosidase activity of sonicated preparations of cultured fibroblasts from a normal subject and those from a patient with Fabry's disease. Heat inactivation of the enzyme in the cell preparation was carried out at 51°C for various periods of time. The heat-inactivated enzymes were then mixed with the substrate in $0.1M$ acetate buffer (pH 5.0), incubated as described in Table 1, with $5\,mM$ substrate and $500\,mM$ inhibitor ($\bullet - \bullet$, α-galactosidase activity of normal cells; $\blacktriangle - \blacktriangle$, of normal cells, myoinositol added; $\bigcirc - \bigcirc$, of cells from patient with Fabry's disease; and $\triangle - \triangle$, of cells from patient, myoinositol added).

References and Notes

1. D. Wise, H. J. Wallace, E. H. Jellinek, *Quart. J. Med.* **31**, 177 (1962).
2. R. O. Brady, A. E. Gal, R. M. Bradley, E. Martensson, A L. Warshaw, L. Laster, *N. Engl. J. Med.* **276**, 1163 (1967).
3. J. A. Kint, *Science* **167**, 1268 (1970).
4. J. T. R. Clarke, J. Knaack, J. C. Crawhall, L. S. Wolfe, *N. Engl. J. Med.* **284**, 233 (1971).
5. C. B. Scharma, *Biochem. Biophys. Res. Commun.* **43**, 572 (1971).
6. E. Beutler and W. Kuhl, *J. Lab. Clin. Med.* **78**, 987 (1971).
7. Supported by Canadian Medical Research Council grant MA 3331. We are grateful to G. Romeo and B. Migeon, who provided us with one cell strain of a patient with Fabry's disease.

Blood Diseases

Double Heterozygous βδ-Thalassemia in Negroes

Leo Zelkowitz, MD; Claudio Torres, MD; Nirmala Bhoopalam, MD; Vincent J. Yakulis; and Paul Heller, MD

The biochemical defect in thalassemia is thought to consist of a diminished capacity of the erythropoietic cells to synthesize one of the polypeptide chains of hemoglobin. Thus, the common variants of this disease have been designated as α- and β-thalassemia. β-Thalassemia is usually associated with a twofold increased proportion of hemoglobin A_2 and a slight elevation of fetal hemoglobin (hemoglobin F) in hemolysates, but many families have been described in which the hemoglobin abnormality is characterized by low or normal levels of hemoglobin A_2 and high concentrations of hemoglobin F (10% to 30%). This variant of the disease has been designated as F-thalassemia or βδ-thalassemia since the synthesis of both β- and δ-chains appears to be impaired. The distribution of hemoglobin F in the erythrocyte population is uneven in contrast to the hereditary persistence of fetal hemoglobin (HPFH) in which all erythrocytes appear to have the same concentration of hemoglobin F.

βδ-Thalassemia has been described in Greeks,[1,2] Italians,[3,4] Turks,[5] Arabs,[6] Negroes,[7,8] and Thais[9,10] and the doubly heterozygous state of β-thalassemia and βδ-thalassemia in individuals of Italian[11-13] and Greek[12-15] origin but not Negroes. The present report deals with this syndrome in the Negro. In addition patients double heterozygous for βδ-thalassemia and an abnormal hemoglobin will be described.

78

Hemoglobin, hematocrit, and red blood cell count measurements were performed. Reticulocyte count; bone marrow examination; determination of serum iron, total iron binding capacity, and bilirubin; and other chemical tests were performed by standard methods.[16]

Blood was collected in sodium edetate and washed three times in 0.9% saline. The washed, packed cells were lysed by addition of an equal volume of distilled water and the stroma removed by centrifugation after the addition of chloroform. The hemoglobin concentration of the hemolysate was adjusted to 10 gm/100 ml by the addition of distilled water.

Hemoglobin F was determined by the method of Singer et al[17] as modified by Betke et al[18] and by electrophoresis in acid agar, pH 6.2,[19] if found elevated by alkali denaturation.

Hemoglobin electrophoresis was performed in cellulose acetate, as described by Kohn[20] and on agar gel in tromethamine (Tris)-edetic acid-boric acid buffer, pH 8.6.[21]

Distribution of fetal hemoglobin in red blood cells was studied by the acid elution method.[22] The distribution of hemoglobin S was determined by the slide elution method.[23]

Hemoglobin A_2 was quantified by anion exchange chromatography[24] or by direct scanning of the unstained agar gel electrophoregram with a densitometer equipped with a 240-mμ filter.

Clinical and Laboratory Findings

Family A.—Patient 1, a 46-year-old Negro man, was admitted to the Veterans Administration West Side Hospital on July 14, 1969, for repair of an indirect left inguinal hernia. The patient had been hospitalized only once, at the age of 21 years, because of a crush injury of the chest. The patient denied any history of blood disease in himself or his family. On the occasion of frequent blood donations (8 to 10 times a year), he was never told of any abnormality.

Physical examination revealed a 3- × 10-cm keloid along the left sternal border and a large indirect left inguinal hernia. The spleen was not palpable but appeared to be enlarged by roentgenographic examination. Findings of the remainder of the physical examination were unremarkable.

The laboratory values and findings were as follows: hemoglobin, 14 gm/100 ml; packed cell volume 45.1%; red blood cell count (RBC) 6.99 × 10⁶/cu mm; white blood cell count (WBC) 10,000/cu mm; mean corpuscular volume (MCV) 64.5 cu μ; mean corpuscular hemoglobin (MCH) 20.1$\mu\mu$g; mean corpuscular hemoglobin concentration (MCHC) 31.2%; reticulocytes, 3%; red blood cells, microcytic and hypochromic with anisocytosis, and poikilocytosis; and several erythrocytes were folded (Fig 1). Total serum bilirubin was 1.7 mg/100 ml with 0.3 mg/100 ml direct; serum iron, 25μg/100 ml; total iron binding capacity (TIBC), 300μg/100 ml; hemoglobin F, 68.0% (acid agar); and hemoglobin A_2, 4.8%. The bone marrow showed erythroid hyperplasia with absent iron stores. Practically all red blood cells contained hemoglobin F but its distribution was uneven (Fig 2).

The hernia was repaired and the patient had an uneventful recovery.

Family studies confirmed the diagnosis of doubly heterozygous $\beta\delta/\beta$-thalassemia in the propositus (Table 1). The father, I-1, and the brother, II-1, of the propositus (Fig 3) are heterozygous for $\beta\delta$-thalassemia, while his son, III-1, carries the gene for β-

79

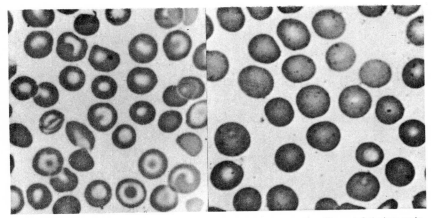

Fig 1.—Peripheral blood smears—family 4. *Left*, heterozygous for $\beta\delta$- and β-thalassemia. *Right*, His brother, who carries the gene for $\beta\delta$-thalassemia (Wright's stain, × 1,000).

Fig 2.—Distribution of hemoglobin F demonstrated by acid elution in patient 1 and his brother. *Left*, $\beta\delta/\beta$-thalassemia, patient 1. *Right*, $\beta\delta$-thalassemia, his brother.

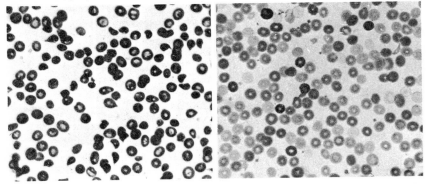

thalassemia.

Family B.—Patient 2, a 24-year-old Negro man was admitted to the Veterans Administration West Side Hospital because of bloody diarrhea of two weeks' duration. A palpable spleen tip was the only significant physical finding. The diagnosis of ulcerative colitis was established by

roentgenographic and proctoscopic examination. The patient responded to medical management and achieved a remission.

The laboratory values and findings were as follows: hemoglobin, 12.3 gm/100 ml; packed cell volume, 38.6% RBC, 5.63 × 10⁶/cu mm, WBC, 9,900/cu mm; MCV, 69 cu μ; MCH

Fig 3.—Pedigree of family A.

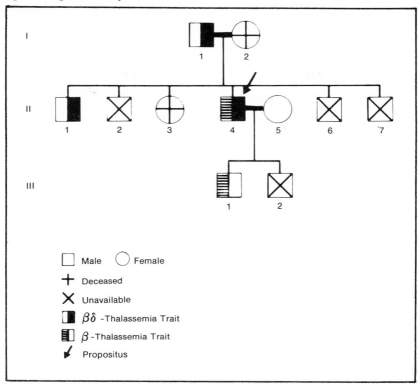

21.8μμg; MCHC, 31.9%; and reticulocytes, 10%. The blood film showed microcytosis, hypochromia, anisocytosis, and poikilocytosis, many target cells, and folded cells. Total serum bilirubin was 1.3 mg/100 ml; serum iron, 75μg/100 ml; TIBC, 260μg/100 ml, hemoglobin F, 72% (acid agar); and hemoglobin A₂, 2.5%.

Family studies proved the presence of the βδ-thalassemia gene in the mother, I-2, and the son, III-1, of the propositus (Table 1 and Fig 4). The father, (I-1), the crucial family member for the demonstration of the β-thalassemia gene, was not available for examination.

Family C.—Patient 3, a 32-year-old Negro male cab driver was admitted to the hospital on Nov 12, 1969, complaining of epigastric pain of two weeks' duration relieved by food. At the age of 21 years, the patient suffered a spontaneous rupture of the spleen which was removed. He was told he had sickle cell anemia at that time.

Findings of physical examination revealed the operative scar and were otherwise unremarkable. Roentgenographic studies revealed a duodenal ulcer. A vagotomy and pyloroplasty

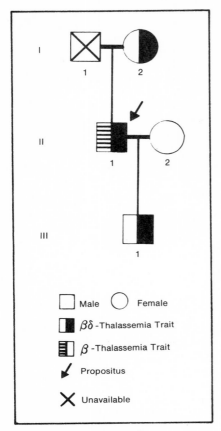

Fig 4.—Pedigree of family B.

☐ Male	◯ Female
◧ βδ-Thalassemia Trait	
▤ β-Thalassemia Trait	
↙ Propositus	
✗ Unavailable	

stippling, Howell-Jolly bodies, and nucleated red blood cells but only rare incompletely sickled cells (Fig 5). The sickle cell preparation and the slide elution test were positive; the bone marrow showed erythroid hyperplasia with increased iron stores. Hemoglobin A_2 was 2.1%; hemoglobin F, 36% (acid agar); hemoglobin S, 61.9%; and hemoglobin A, absent. Hemoglobin F was unequally distributed, as was hemoglobin S.

The patient's father was found to have hemoglobin C in combination with βδ-thalassemia. Neither the propositus nor his father produced hemoglobin A (Table 2 and Fig 6). The patient's father (I-1) carried the gene for βδ-thalassemia and hemoglobin C while his mother (I-2) had sickle cell trait. His wife (II-2) carried the gene for β-thalassemia but did not transmit it. The βδ-thalassemia gene was inherited by two children (III-1 and III-4) and the other two children (III-2 and III-3) inherited the sickle cell gene.

Because the patient's hemoglobin F level was so much higher than that of the children with βδ-thalassemia trait, the possibility that the hemoglobin S carrying red blood cells with the smallest amount of hemoglobin F were more rapidly destroyed than those with a larger proportion of hemoglobin F was considered. Blood was obtained from the patient and the reticulocyte-rich layer was separated after centrifugation at 100,000 × g for one hour. Hemoglobin F concentration was determined in the top (reticulocyte-rich) and bottom (reticulocyte-poor) layer of the packed red blood cells. The top layer contained 21% alkaline-resistant hemoglobin

was performed. The patient's recovery was delayed by pneumonitis and would dehiscence which required surgical repair.

The laboratory values and findings were as follows: hemoglobin, 15.9 gm/100 ml; packed cell volume, 49%; RBC, 5.12 × 10^6/cu mm; WBC, 9,500/cu mm; MCV, 96 cu μ; MCH, 31.0$\mu\mu$g; MCHC, 32.4%; and reticulocytes, 3%. Peripheral blood picture showed anisocytosis, poikilocytosis, target cells, folded cells, basophilic

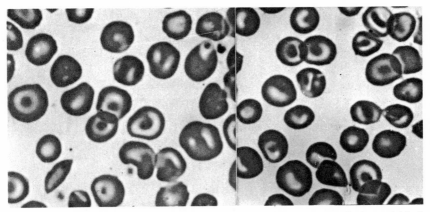

Fig 5.—Peripheral blood smears—family C. *Left,* Patient 3, heterozygous for hemoglobin S and $\beta\delta$-thalassemia. *Right,* His father, heterozygous for hemoglobin C and $\beta\delta$-thalassemia (Wright's stain × 1,000).

and the bottom layer, 28%, which suggests that the older cells had a higher content of hemoglobin F.

The mean level of hemoglobin F determined by alkali denaturation in the six simple heterozygotes for $\beta\delta$-thalassemia identified in this present study was 21.1%. This exceeds the mean level observed in 86 Greek simple heterozygotes for $\beta\delta$-thalassemia who had 10.9% hemoglobin F.[15]

Comment

The patients 1 and 2, apparently the first Negroes described with $\beta\delta/\beta$ thalassemia, had a milder clinical picture than the 21 patients with $\beta\delta/\beta$-thalassemia of Greek origin reported by Stamatoyannopoulos et al.[15] These patients had splenomegaly and elevated bilirubin levels, even those

without anemia. Their mean hemoglobin level was 9.9 gm/100 ml (range 5.3 to 13.1 gm/100 ml) and nine patients required transfusions. The patients of this report also had enlarged spleens and elevated bilirubin levels but were not anemic and were otherwise asymptomatic. The morphologic changes of their red blood cells were similar to those described in Greeks.[15] Both patients completed military duty without any problems related to their hematologic status.

The study of Comings and Motulsky[25] demonstrated the complete absence of normal δ-chain production in an individual with $\beta\delta$-thalassemia heterozygous for hemoglobin A_2 ($\alpha_2\delta_2^{16\ \text{gly}\rightarrow\text{arg}}$) which suggests that the δ-gene in the cis position to the gene for $\beta\delta$-thalassemia was completely inactive. It therefore appears

Fig 6.—Pedigree of family C.

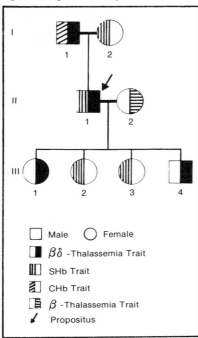

Male □   Female ○

◧ βδ-Thalassemia Trait

Ⅲ SHb Trait

◩ CHb Trait

⊟ β-Thalassemia Trait

↙ Propositus

that the elevation of hemoglobin A₂ in patients with βδ/β-thalassemia, if increased, is the product of the δ-gene in the cis position to the β-thalassemia gene. Of 28 doubly heterozygous individuals of Mediterranean origin, only one had an elevated hemoglobin A₂ level.[11-15] The normal level of hemoglobin A₂ in our patient 2, therefore, does not exclude double heterozygosity. It just suggests that the δ-gene in cis with β-thalassemia is variable in its expression.

Observation of the distribution of hemoglobin F within the red blood cell population is the most valuable way to distinguish βδ-thalassemia from HPFH since the distribution of hemoglobin F is homogeneous in HPFH and heterogeneous in βδ-thalassemia. If, however, the level of hemoglobin F is very high as in patients 1 and 2, almost all the erythrocytes contain hemoglobin F which may make it difficult to demonstrate unevenness of distribution. Family studies are therefore required to establish the diagnosis with certainty.

The study of Pearson[8] and our present observation suggest that the combination of βδ-thalassemia and hemoglobin S produces fewer symptoms than the homozygous state of sickle cell anemia. This protective effect is believed to be due to the failure of hemoglobin F to interact with hemoglobin S[26] which accounts for the absence of sickled cells in the peripheral blood of our patient. This diminished sickling tendency may have prevented the autosplenectomy so common in adults with sickle cell anemia and may have maintained splenic enlargement in patient 3 resulting in the spontaneous rupture of his enlarged spleen. This explanation is consistent with the observation of Serjeant[27] who noted that splenomegaly and a decreased number of irreversibly sickled cells was more frequently observed in patients with sickle cell anemia with high levels of hemoglobin F. The higher level of alkali-resistant hemoglobin in the propositus of family F than in two of his children with βδ-thalassemia trait may be due to the more rapid destruction of those red blood cells containing the least amount of hemoglobin F. This explanation is supported by the observation of Gabuzda et al, who noted a higher proportion of hemo-

Table 1.—Hematologic Data—Families A and B

| | Age (yr) | Sex | Hemoglobin (gm/100 ml) | Mean Corpuscular Volume (cu μ) | Morphology | Hemoglobin A_2 (%) | Hemoglobin F | | |
							Alkali Denaturation (%)	Acid Agar (%)	Distribution
Family A									
I-1	78	M	13.2	85	+	2.6	19.0	35.0	Uneven
II-1	52	M	14.7	87	+	2.3	21.0	33.3	Uneven
II-4*	46	M	14.1	64.5	+++†	4.8	54.0	68.0	Uneven
II-5	38	M	12.2	99	0	1.5	0.7	...	...
III-1	18	M	12.0	87	+	4.5	1.7	...	...
Family B									
I-2	47	F	13.7	89	+	2.1	15.3	35.0	Uneven
II-1*	24	M	12.3	69	+++	2.5	52.0	72.0	Uneven
II-2	22	F	12.3	88	0	2.4	0.9	...	...
III-1	15	M	10.5	64	++	2.2	24.3	42.8	Uneven

* Propositus.
† Patient also had iron deficiency.

Table 2.—Hematologic Data—Family C

| | Age (yr) | Sex | Hemoglobin (gm/100 ml) | Mean Corpuscular Volume (cu μ) | Morphology | Hemoglobin S (%) | Hemoglobin A_2 (%) | Hemoglobin F* | |
								(%)	Distribution
I-1	68	M	14.7	80.5	++++	...	73.9†	26.1	Uneven
I-2	65	F	13.2	89	0	40	2.0	0.7	...
II-1‡	38	M	15.9	96	++++	61.9	2.1	28.3	Uneven
II-2	35	F	12.5	75	+	...	4.6	2.3	...
III-1	17	F	14.9	86.1	+	...	1.8	23.8	Uneven
III-2	15	F	12.2	81.1	0	40	1.8	0.8	...
III-3	12	F	13.7	86.7	0	40	2.2	1.1	...
III-4	4	M	13.0	85.4	+	...	2.5	23.4	Uneven

* Hemoglobin F determined by alkali denaturation.
† Hemoglobins A_2 + C.
‡ Propositus.

85

globin F in older cells of patients with thalassemia.[28]

The findings described by Pearson[8] are similar to those in our family C. No hemoglobin A was present in the double heterozygotes for $\beta\delta$-thalassemia and hemoglobin S, which suggests that in this condition, as in HPFH, there appears to be complete suppression of both β- and δ-globin chain synthesis in the cis position.

The difference in hemoglobin F levels between Negro and Greek patients with $\beta\delta$-thalassemia is similar to the differences noted in these two populations with HPFH.[29,30] Greeks with HPFH have 14.5% hemoglobin F[29] while Negroes have 25.65%.[30] It would appear reasonable to assume that when the β- and δ-genes are suppressed, the Negro is capable of greater γ-chain production which results in higher levels of hemoglobin F.

This may be a manifestation of the heterogeneity of thalassemia or an expression of the genetic difference between these two populations which results in an altered phenotypic expression of identical genetic defects.

Summary

The clinical, hematologic, and genetic findings in three black families with $\beta\delta$-thalassemia are described. Double heterozygosity for β-and $\beta\delta$-thalassemia, or for $\beta\delta$-thalassemia and hemoglobin S or C was found to produce only mild disease characterized by compensated hemolysis, hyperbilirubinemia, and splenomegaly. The level of fetal hemoglobin in Negroes with $\beta\delta$-thalassemia is higher than in similarly affected Greeks.

References

1. Malamos B, Fessas P, Stamatoyannopoulos G: Types of thalassemia-trait carriers as revealed by a study of their incidence in Greece. *Brit J Haemat* **8:**5-14, 1962.
2. Stamatoyannopoulos G, Papayannopoulou T, Fessas P, et al: The beta-delta thalassemias. *Ann NY Acad Sci* **165:**25-36, 1969.
3. Silvestroni E, Bianco I, Reitano G: Three cases of homozygous $\beta\delta$-thalassemia (or microcythaemia) with high haemoglobin F in a Sicilian family. *Acta Haemat* **40:**220-229, 1968.
4. Brancati C, Baglioni C: Homozygous $\beta\delta$ thalassemia ($\beta\delta$ microcythaemia). *Nature* **212:**262-264, 1966.
5. Aksoy M, Erdem S: Some problems of hemoglobin patterns in different thalassemic syndromes showing the heterogeneity of beta-thalassemia genes. *Ann NY Acad Sci* **165:**13-14, 1969.
6. Ramot B, Ben-Bassat I, Gafni D, et al: A family with three $\beta\delta$-thalassemia homozygotes. *Blood* **35:**158-165, 1970.

7. Weatherall DJ: Biochemical phenotypes of thalassemia in the American Negro population. *Ann NY Acad Sci* **119:**450-462, 1964.
8. Pearson HA: Hemoglobin S-thalassemia syndrome in Negro children. *Ann NY Acad Sci* **165:**83-92, 1969.
9. Wasi P, Na-Nakorn S, Pootrakul S, et al: Alpha- and beta-thalassemia in Thailand. *Ann NY Acad Sci* **165:**60-82, 1969.
10. Flatz G, Pik C, Sringam S: Haemoglobinopathies in Thailand: II. Incidence and distribution of elevations of hemoglobin A_2 and hemoglobin F: A survey of 2,790 people. *Brit J Haemat* **11:**227-236, 1965.
11. Zuelzer WW, Robinson AR, Booker CR: Reciprocal relationship of hemoglobins A_2 and F in beta chain thalassemias: A key to the genetic control of hemaglobulin F. *Blood* **17:**393-408, 1961.
12. Necheles TF, Allen DM, Gerald PS: The many forms of thalassemia: Definition and classification of the thalassemia syndromes. *Ann*

NY Acad Sci 165:5-12, 1969.

13. Wolff JA, Ignatov VG: Heterogeneity of thalassemia major. Amer J Dis Child 105:234-242, 1963.

14. Gabuzda TG, Nathan DG, Gardner FH: Thalassemia trait: Genetic combinations of increased fetal and A₂ hemoglobins. New Eng J Med 270:1212-1217, 1964.

15. Stamatoyannopoulos G, Fessas P, Papayannopoulou T: F-thalassemia a study of 31 families with simple heterozygotes and combinations of F-thalassemia with A₂-thalassemia. Amer J Med 47:194-208, 1969.

16. Page LB, Culver PJ (eds): A Syllabus of Laboratory Examinations in Clinical Diagnosis. Cambridge, Mass, Harvard University Press, 1961.

17. Singer K, Chernoff AI, Singer L: Studies on abnormal hemoglobins: I. Their demonstration in sickle cell anemia and other hematologic disorders by means of alkali denaturation. Blood 6:413-428, 1951.

18. Betke K, Marti HR, Schlicht I: Estimation of small percentages of foetal hemoglobin. Nature 184:1877-1878, 1959.

19. Robinson AR, Robson M, Harrison AP, et al: A new technique for differentiation of hemoglobin. J Lab Clin Med 50:745-752, 1957.

20. Kohn J: Separation of haemoglobins on cellulose acetate. J Clin Path 22:109-111, 1969.

21. Josephson AM, Weinstein G, Yakulis VJ, et al: A new variant of hemoglobin M disease: Hemoglobin M Chicago. J Lab Clin Med 59:918-925, 1962.

22. Shepard MK, Weatherall DJ, Conley CL: Semi-quantitative estimation of the distribution of fetal hemoglobin in red cell populations. Bull Hopkins Hosp 110:293-310, 1962.

23. Yakulis VJ, Heller P: An elution test for the visualization of hemoglobin S in blood smears. Blood 24:198-201, 1964.

24. Huisman TH, Dozy AM: Studies on the heterogeneity of hemoglobins: IX. The use of Tris (hydroxymethyl)-aminomethane^{HCl} buffers in the anion-exchange chromatography of hemoglobins. J Chromatogr 19:160-169, 1965.

25. Comings DE, Motulsky AG: Absence of cis delta chain synthesis in (βδ) thalassemia (F-thalassemia). Blood 28:54-69, 1966.

26. Heller P: Hemoglobinopathic dysfunction of the red cell. Amer J Med 41:799-814, 1966.

27. Serjeant GR: Irreversibly sickled cells and splenomegaly in sickle-cell anaemia. Brit J Haemat 19:635-641, 1970.

28. Gabuzda TG, Nathan DG, Gardner FH: The turnover of hemoglobins A, F and A₂ in the peripheral blood of three patients with thalassemia. J Clin Invest 42:1678-1688, 1963.

29. Fessas P, Stamatoyannopoulos G: Hereditary persistence of fetal hemoglobin: A study and a comparison. Blood 24:223-240, 1964.

30. Conley CL, Weatherall DJ, Richardson SN, et al: Hereditary persistence of fetal hemoglobin: A study of 79 affected persons in 15 Negro families in Baltimore. Blood 21:261-281, 1963.

Cross-reacting material in genetic variants of haemophilia B

DOMINIQUE MEYER, ETHEL BIDWELL, AND MARIE JOSÉ LARRIEU

Genetic variants of haemophilia A and B (factor VIII and IX deficiencies) have been recently demonstrated by the ability or inability of the patient's plasma to neutralize specific human antibodies against factor VIII or IX (Roberts, Gross, Webster, and Dejanov, 1966; Denson, Biggs, and Mannucci, 1968; Hoyer and Breckenridge, 1968; Roberts, Grizzle, Mc-Lester, and Penick, 1968; Feinstein, Chong, Kasper, and Rapaport, 1969; Denson, Biggs, Haddon, Borrett, and Cobb, 1969; Brown, Hougie, and Roberts, 1970; Meyer, Dray, and Larrieu, 1970; Hoyer and Breckenridge, 1970; Meyer and Larrieu, 1971). In most patients (haemophilia A⁻ or B⁻) immunological cross-reacting material was absent, while in 10 to 15% of them an inactive protein could be demonstrated (haemophilia A⁺ or B⁺). However, conflicting data were obtained in haemophilia A when using factor VIII antibodies raised in different species (rabbit, goat) by immunization with partially purified factor VIII. Depending on the reactivity of the various antibodies, inactive cross-reacting material could be demonstrated in a highly variable percentage of haemophilia A patients: 100% (Zimmerman, Ratnoff, and Powell, 1971; Stites, Hershgold, Perlman, and Fudenberg, 1971; Meyer, Lavergne, Larrieu, and Josso, 1972), 90% (Bennett and Huehns, 1970), or around 15% (Denson *et al*, 1969; Gralnick, Abrell, and Bagley, 1971). The present study demonstrates a similar discrepancy when the reactivity of different haemophilia B plasmas was compared with two types of factor IX antibodies, namely, a human inhibitor which occurred in a transfused haemophilia B patient, and rabbit antibodies raised by immunization with a partially purified antigen.

Materials and Methods

The factor IX concentrate used as a source of antigen was a sample from a batch of human material (RD40) prepared at the Oxford Haemophilia Centre by batch adsorption on DEAE-cellulose followed by displacement elution in a column (Dike, Bidwell, and Rizza, 1972). This concentrate contained 62 U/ml factor IX, 50 U/ml factor II, 44 U/ml factor X, and a very low concentration of factor VII (1·7 U/ml). The protein concentration was 10 mg/ml and the purification with respect to factor IX was 400-fold.

Rabbit antisera were obtained by injection of equal parts of factor IX concentrate and complete Freund's adjuvant. Three injections (6 mg protein) were given at intervals of eight days, the first one in the popliteal lymph node and subsequent ones in foot pads. Blood was drawn 10 days after the last injection, and allowed to clot in glass tubes, which were kept at 37° C for six hours and at 4°C for 12 hours. Serum was obtained by centrifugation at 5000 *g* for 15 min, oxalated, adsorbed with barium carbonate (40 mg/ml), and heated at 56°C for 30 minutes. The antibody titres (Denson, 1967) were 5 U/ml and 18 U/ml (1 U was defined as the amount of serum destroying 75% factor IX after incubation at 37°C for 15 min). The anti-factor II and anti-factor X antibody titres were < 2 U/ml. These antibodies were not specific for factor IX, as by immunodiffusion four lines of precipitation were shown against normal plasma or factor IX concentrate.

Human factor IX antibody was a specific inhibitor which appeared in a haemophilia B patient after multiple transfusions. The antibody titre was 15 U/ml

Factor IX activity was measured by a one-stage assay (Langdell, Wagner, and Brinkhous, 1953), and prothrombin time with human and ox-brain thromboplastin (Thrombotest) as previously described (Meyer and Larrieu, 1971).

Inhibitor-neutralizing activity was measured by a modified two-stage procedure (Denson *et al*, 1969). In the first step, 0·4 ml of normal or test plasma was incubated at 37°C for 15 min with 0·1 ml of an appropriate dilution of human or rabbit antibody. In the second step, 0·2 ml of normal plasma was added to an equal volume of the first mixture. After a second incubation at 37°C for 15 min residual factor IX was measured by a one-stage assay. Results were expressed as units of neutralized inhibitor.

Results

INHIBITOR-NEUTRALIZING ACTIVITY IN CONTROL PLASMAS

The specificity of the factor IX assays ensures the specificity of the inhibitor-neutralizing technique for the antigenic determinants of factor IX. Other coagulation factor antibodies, such as anti-factor VIII (from human or rabbit origin) or rabbit anti-human factor II,[1] tested in the same system, did not interfere with the final assay of factor IX after the two incubations.

Inhibitor-neutralizing activity was measured in normal plasma (38 experiments): it varied from 0·85 to 1·07 unit (mean 1·03 ± 0·07 unit) when using

[1]Kindly provided by J. M. Lavergne and F. Josso, Hôpital Necker, Paris.

human antibody (Fig. 1), and from 0·85 to 1·25 unit (mean 0·92 ± 0.05 unit) when using antihuman factor IX antiserum (Fig. 2). Cross-reacting material was present in normal serum as well as in the plasma of coagulation deficiencies other than factor IX. It was lacking in aluminium hydroxide or barium sulphate-adsorbed plasma or serum, the results being the same as those with citrated saline.

INHIBITOR-NEUTRALIZING ACTIVITY IN PATIENTS WITH HAEMOPHILIA B

Twenty-two haemophilia B patients were tested in the same way using both human and rabbit antibodies.

Human antibody

Plasma samples from 13 haemophilia B patients failed to neutralize the human antibody. These patients were classified as haemophilia B⁻. Five plasmas contained an amount of cross-reacting material identical to that in normal plasma, and four showed intermediate results (Fig. 1). These nine patients were classified as haemophilia B⁺.

Rabbit antiserum

The capacity of the same plasmas to neutralize the rabbit antihuman factor IX antibodies appeared entirely different. Only one patient out of the 22 tested lacked immunologically detectable crossreacting material (Fig. 2). This patient had a moderate form of haemophilia B (factor IX activity 4%). In 14 patients plasma inhibitor neutralizing activity varied from 0·65 to 1·1 unit, ie, within the normal

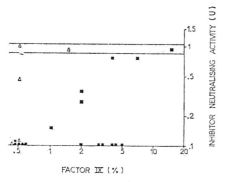

Fig. 1 *Inhibitor-neutralizing activity in 22 cases of haemophilia B (human factor IX inhibitor)*

■ Haemophilia B   △ Haemophilia B_M

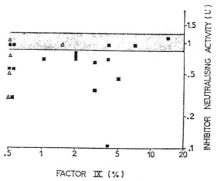

Fig. 2 *Inhibitor-neutralizing activity in 22 cases of haemophilia B (rabbit factor IX antiserum).*

▨ Normal range.

range, and seven patients had intermediate values, from 0·30 to 0·55 unit. The same results were observed using two different rabbit antisera. No correlation was found between the level of active factor IX and the amount of factor IX antigen.

OX BRAIN CLOTTING TIME IN PATIENTS WITH HAEMOPHILIA B
In five of the 22 patients tested, the Thrombotest time (or clotting time in the presence of ox-brain thromboplastin) was prolonged on repeated testing (62-85 sec) while the clotting time was normal in the presence of human brain thromboplastin. These patients were classified as haemophilia B_M (Hougie and Twomey, 1967). Cross-reacting material was present in three of these patients when tested by human antibody, and in all five when tested with rabbit antibody (Table I).

Factor IX Activity %	Factor IX Antigen (INA Units)	
	Human Antibody	Rabbit Antibody
< 1	0	0·50
< 1	0	0·30
< 1	0·46	1·05
< 1	1·05	0·95
1·5	0·92	0·95
Control (mean)	0·92	1·03

Table I *Inhibitor-neutralizing activity in haemophilia B_M (five patients) (comparison of two types of antibodies)*

RELATIONSHIP BETWEEN FACTOR IX VARIANTS
Among the 22 patients with haemophilia B we studied with both methods, four groups could be distinguished when using factor IX human antibody (Table II). In the first group (11 patients with a severe or a moderate form of the disease), the Thrombotest was normal and antigenic activity lacking. In the second group (six patients with moderate haemophilia), the Thrombotest was normal, and the plasma

Antibody	No. of Cases	Haemophilia	
		B_M	B^+
Human			
I	11	—	—
II	6	—	+
III	2	+	—
IV	3	+	+
Rabbit			
I	1	—	—
II	16	—	+
III	0	+	—
IV	5	+	+

Table II *Classification of patients with haemophilia B according to the results of Thrombotest and inhibitor-neutralizing activity*

contained factor IX antigenic determinants. Conversely in the third group (two patients with severe haemophilia) the Thrombotest was prolonged but antigenic material lacking. In the fourth group, three patients had both haemophilia B_M and B^+. The groups were entirely different when employing rabbit antibody (Table II). Twenty-one patients were classified in groups II and IV (haemophilia B^+), and one in group I.

Discussion

A large heterogeneity with a wide spectrum of variants had already been demonstrated in haemophilia B when using a human factor IX inhibitor. Two different molecular abnormalities have been recently described: haemophilia B_M (Hougie and Twomey, 1967) and haemophilia B^+ (Denson et al, 1968; Roberts et al, 1968; Meyer and Larrieu, 1971). Our results, obtained with factor IX antisera raised in rabbits, suggest that in nearly all haemophilia B patients (21 out of 22), the lack of factor IX activity is due to the synthesis of an inactive protein, having antigenic determinants in common with normal factor IX. These results are in agreement with those obtained with factor VIII antibodies raised in rabbits (Zimmerman et al, 1971; Bennett and Huehns, 1970; Stites et al, 1971; Meyer et al, 1972). The large discrepancy between the results obtained with the two types of factor IX antibodies in haemophilia B patients suggests that more than one antigenic site is involved on factor IX protein. Factor IX antisera raised in rabbits probably contain some antibodies which react with antigenic determinants present on the factor IX molecule, other than those responsible for the development of antibody(ies) in some haemophilia B patients after multiple transfusions.

This work was supported by a grant from INSERM. We wish to thank G. W. R. Dike (Oxford Haemophilia Centre) for providing factor IX concentrate. The technical help of B. Obert is gratefully acknowledged.

References

Bennett, E., and Huehns, E. R. (1970). Immunological differentiation of three types of haemophilia and identification of some female carriers. Lancet, 2, 956-958.
Brown, P. E., Hougie, C., and Roberts, H. R. (1970). The genetic heterogeneity of haemophilia B. New Engl. J. Med., 283, 61-64.
Denson, K. W. E. (1967). The Use of Antibodies in the Study of Blood Coagulation. vol. 1, p. 244. Blackwell, Oxford and Edinburgh.
Denson, K. W. E., Biggs, R., and Mannucci, P. M. (1968). An investigation of three patients with Christmas disease due to an abnormal type of factor IX. J. clin. Path., 21, 160-165.
Denson, K. W. E., Biggs, R., Haddon, M. E., Borrett, R., and Cobb, K. (1969). Two types of haemophilia (A⁺ and A⁻): a study of 48 cases. Brit. J. Haemat., 17, 163-171.
Dike, G. W. R., Bidwell, E., and Rizza, C. R. (1972). The preparation

and clinical use of a new concentrate containing Factor IX, prothrombin, and Factor X. *Brit. J. Haemat.*, in press.

Feinstein, D., Chong, M. N. Y., Kasper, C. K., and Rapaport, S. I. (1969). Haemophilia A: polymorphism detectable by a Factor VIII antibody. *Science*, 163, 1071-1072.

Gralnick, H. R., Abrell, E., and Bagley, J. (1971). Immunological studies of factor VIII (anti-haemophiliac globulin) in haemophilia A. *Nature [New Biol.]*, 230, 16-17.

Hougie, C., and Twomey, J. J. (1967). Haemophilia B$_M$: a new type of Factor IX deficiency. *Lancet*, 1, 698-700.

Hoyer, L. W., and Breckenridge, R. T. (1968). Immunological studies of antihemophilic factor (AHF, factor-VIII): cross-reacting material in a genetic variant of haemophilia A. *Blood*, 32, 962-971.

Hoyer, L. W., and Breckenridge, T. R. (1970). Immunologic studies of antihemophilic factor (AHF, factor-VIII). II. Properties of cross-reacting material. *Blood*, 35, 809-820.

Langdell, R. D., Wagner, R. H., and Brinkhous, K. M. (1953). Effect of antihemophilic factor on one stage clotting tests. *J. Lab clin. Med.*, 41, 637-647.

Meyer, D., Dray, L., and Larrieu, M. J. (1970). Hémophilie. Les variants des Facteurs VIII et IX. *Nouv. Rev. franç. Hémat.*, 10, 619-626.

Meyer, D., and Larrieu, M. J. (1971). Factor VIII and IX variants. Relationship between haemophilia B$_M$ and haemophilia B$^+$. *Europ. J. clin. Invest.*, 1, 425-431.

Meyer, D., Lavergne, J. M., Larrieu, M. J., and Josso, F. (1972). Cross-reacting material in congenital factor VIII deficiencies (haemophilia A and von Willebrand's disease). *Thrombos. Res.*, in press.

Roberts, H. R., Grizzle, J. E., McLester, W. D., and Penick, G. D. (1968). Genetic variants of Hemophilia B: detection by means of a specific PTC inhibitor. *J. clin. Invest.*, 47, 360-365.

Roberts, H. R., Gross, G. P., Webster, W. P., Dejanov, I. I., and Penick, G. D. (1966). Acquired inhibitors of plasma Factor IX. A study of their induction, properties and neutralisation. *Amer. J. med. Sci.*, 251, 43-50 and 56.

Stites, D. P., Hershgold, E. J., Perlman, J. D., and Fudenberg, H. H. (1971). Factor VIII detection by hemagglutination inhibition: hemophilia A and Von Willebrand's disease. *Science*, 171, 196-197.

Zimmerman, T. S., Ratnoff, O. D., and Powell, A. E. (1971). Immunologic differentiation of classic hemophilia (factor VIII deficiency) and von Willebrand's disease. *J. clin. Invest.*, 50, 244-254.

91

Other Disorders

C1r Deficiency: an Inborn Error
Associated with Cutaneous and Renal Disease

N. K. Day, H. Geiger, R. Stroud, M. deBracco, B. Mancado, D. Windhorst, and R. A. Good

INTRODUCTION

In recent years, progress has been made in the purification of the subcomponents of C1, C1q, C1r, and C1s, and it is now possible to study the relationship of these subcomponents to the complement system and to each other, and to clarify their physiology and role in disease. Patients deficient in C1 have been described by several investigators. Among these, patients having deficiencies of each subcomponent of C1-C1q (1-3), C1r (4), and C1s (5) have been described.

Recently we have studied two patients, a brother and a sister, who have a deficiency of C1r.[1] The brother (18 yr old) has had clinical manifestations resembling lupus erythematosus for 5 yr. At the age of 13, he developed erythematosus, scaling atrophic lesions which slowly

---

[1] Mancado, B., N. K. B. Day, R. A. Good, and D. Windhorst. Lupus erythematosus-like syndrome associated with a familial defect of the first component of complement. *N. Engl. J. Med.* **286**: 689.

progressed to involve the skin of his nose, around his ears, and on the upper part of his chest and back and upper extremities. At the age of 16, he was hospitalized three times for acute episodes characterized by high fever, nausea, vomiting, exacerbation of skin lesions, and swelling and stiffness of wrists, elbows, and knees. He had normal renal function, negative lupus erythematosus (L.E.) tests and no antinuclear antibodies, but total serum complement was low. A kidney biopsy performed at the age of 17 is reported to have shown focal membranous glomerulitis in one of eight glomeruli, and was interpreted as early renal involvement with lupus erythematosus.

The sister (24 yr old) had recurrent attacks of otitis media and upper respiratory tract infections since infancy and early childhood, but now has arthralgia and recurrent episodes of rhinobronchitis. Three siblings have died. One brother died at age 12 with "lupus erythematosus," described by the mother as being similar to the disease of the male patient studied here. Two other siblings died in infancy, one with gastroenteritis and one of unknown cause. Studies of hemolytic serum complement and complement components in both patients indicated extremely low total hemolytic complement and C1. Extensive studies of the sera of these patients are reported in this paper. These studies show that C1r is undetectable in the serum immunochemically, and that upon addition of purified C1r to the serum, hemolytic C1 activity is restored. No evidence of a deficiency of hemolytic C1 was detectable in the sera of the investigated family members (parents and three siblings). The sera of these patients provide a useful basis for the study of the dependence of known complement biologic activities of C1r. It is shown that the later complement components can be activated in the absence of C1r. These findings support the view that an alternative pathway for activation of the terminal portion of the complement cascade exists which does not utilize the conventional pathway through the usual early components.

METHODS

Buffers for complement assays. The disodium salt of ethylenediaminetetraacetic acid (EDTA),[2] reagent grade

---

[2] *Abbreviations used in this paper:* CVF, Cobra venom factor; EDTA, ethylenediaminetetraacetic acid; EA, sensitized erythrocytes; BSA, bovine serum albumin; LPS, lipopolysaccharide.

Na$_2$H$_2$EDTA, was titrated to pH 7.4 at a stock concentration of 0.15 mole/liter. Na$_2$MgEDTA (Geigy Chemical Corp., Ardsley, N. Y.) was also titrated to pH 7.4 at a stock concentration of 0.15 mole/liter. Gelatin Veronal buffer and glucose gelatin Veronal buffer with and without Ca^{++} and Mg^{++} (GGV^{++}, GGV^{--}) were prepared as described previously (6).

Human serum. Blood was allowed to clot for 1 hr at room temperature. The serum was removed after centrifugation at 4°C, aliquoted, and stored at −70° until used.

Human C1 subcomponents C1q, C1r, C1s, and antisera. C1q, C1r, and C1s and their respective antisera were prepared and purified as described previously (7–10).

Guinea pig C2. Partially purified C2 was prepared from guinea pig serum (Texas Biological Laboratory Inc., Fort Worth, Tex.) according to the method described by Nelson et al. (11).

EAC1, EAC1,4, EAC4. Cell intermediates with C1 were prepared according to methods described previously (12, 13).

Assays of total complement (CH50) and of the complement components. Sensitization of erythrocytes from sheep (6) and the measurement of total complement in 50% hemolytic units (CH50) were carried out as previously described (14).

Assays of human C1, C4, C2, and C3 complex were determined according to methods described before (12).

Assay of human C3, C5, C6, C7, C8, and C9. Functionally pure complement components for the assays of these components and EAC1gp4-7 human for use in assay of C8 and C9 were obtained from Cordis Laboratories and the assays were carried out according to the method described by Nelson, Jensen, Gigli, and Tamura (11). The percentage experimental error of the C components 1–9 ranged between 5% and 10%.

Assay of C1 subcomponents, C1q, C1r, and C1s and C1-esterase inhibitor. C1q was assayed by the Mancini technique (15). Antibody to this component was prepared by the method described by Morse and Christian (10) or by the method of Yonemasu and Stroud (7) with equivalent results.

C1r was measured by Ouchterlony immunodiffusion in 1% agarose, using monospecific antiserum (8).

C1s was measured according to the method of Nagaki and Stroud (16).

C1-esterase inhibitor was assayed by the Mancini method. The results are expressed as a percentage of the value in a normal serum pool.

Endotoxin lipopolysaccharide (LPS). Salmonella typhosa batch 225323 from Difco was dissolved in isotonic saline. A dose response experiment was previously set up to determine the optimum amount of LPS required to fix a maximum amount of hemolytic complement. To a constant volume of normal serum, varying concentrations of endotoxin were added, and the CH50 and C3 determined after incubation. This amount of endotoxin was then added to the test serum. Controls consisting of serum and saline and a normal pool of serum and LPS were included. The tubes were incubated at 37°C, for 15 min and centrifuged at 16,000 rpm, and then C1q, C1, C4, C2, C3, C5, C6, C7, C8, and C9 were assayed.

Purified cobra venom factor. Purified cobra venom factor (CVF) was prepared and assayed as described earlier (17). Test serum and control sera were incubated with equal volumes of CVF at 37°C for 1 hr and all the complement components were then measured.

Bovine serum albumin (BSA) anti-BSA complexes. BSA rabbit anti-BSA complexes were prepared at equivalence as described (18). The experiment was set up with one volume of the complex suspended in saline to two parts of the patient's serum. Controls consisted of patients' serum and saline. Normal serum and immune complex and normal serum with saline were also set up. All the complement components were then measured.

Immune adherence was measured according to the method of Nishioka (19).

Bactericidal activity was measured according to the method of Muschel and Treffers (20), using a rough (Lilly) strain of *Escherichia coli.*

RESULTS

Table I represents comparisons of total complement (CH-50) and each of the separate complement components of the deficient brother and sister and of all the other family members with a series of values from 40 healthy adults 20-40 yr of age. While total hemolytic complement activity was not detectable at any concentration in the sera of the two patients, the rest of the family members (parents, one brother, and two sisters) had elevated levels. C1 was markedly depressed in the brother and sister (37 and 2,533 CH50 U/ml, respectively, compared to the normal 430,000 U/ml). C4 was markedly elevated in the sister's serum. The remaining C components in sera from the rest of the family members were variable. However, C8 seemed to be constantly elevated in all the family members. Because of the marked deficiency of C1 in the patients' sera, further analysis of the subcomponents of C1 were undertaken. Table II represents the results of C1q, C1r, C1s, and C1-esterase inhibitor measured by immunodiffusion using monospecific antisera. The values of C1q expressed as micrograms per milliliter were normal in both the brother and sister. Radial immunodiffusion assay of recently isolated C1r (9) cannot yet be expressed in units, but by the Ouchterlony method of immunodiffusion and by immunoelectrophoresis no bands were produced with patient serum against monospecific anti-C1r Fig. 1). C1s expressed as micrograms protein per milliter was reduced to 30–40% of normal in the serum of both patients. C1-esterase inhibitor activity was greater than normal in the sister.

97

TABLE I

Total Hemolytic C and C Components in C1r-Deficient Patients and Healthy Family Members

	CH50	C1	C4	C2	C3	C5	C6	C7	C8	C9
Patients										
Brother	<12*	37*	401,800§	876	4,500‖	9,000‖	9,400‖	9,000‖	92,000§	28,000‖
Sister	<12*	2,533*	2,460,000‖	1100	7,800‖	9,800‖	7,200	6,600	78,000	21,000§
Family										
Mother	106‖	512,000	105,128‡	1960§	3,100	3,400	7,200	5,600	160,000‖	15,000
Father	109‖	318,000	133,333‡	1560	2,700	6,000‖	6,400	11,000‖	115,000‖	13,000
Brother, E.	95‖	390,000	262,564	1300	3,700‖	3,800	8,800‖	7,200§	110,000‖	28,000‖
Sister, R. M.	95‖	350,000	148,718	1600	3,800‖	3,100	5,500	6,600	190,000‖	20,000
Sister, M.	78‖	360,000	207,692	1320	2,400	2,600	4,800‡	5,400	128,000‖	14,000
Normal										
X̄¶	45	430,000	246,000	1350	2,600	3,415	6,150	5,529	65,889	15,795
1S**	37–53	286,000–574,000	144,500–347,500	850–1850	2,068–3,132	2,595–4,235	5,059–7,241	4,094–6,964	46,311–85,467	9,946–20,644
2S‡‡	29–61	145,000–721,000	43,000–449,000	350–2350	1,536–3,664	1,775–5,055	3,968–8,332	2,659–8,399	26,733–105,045	4,097–27,493

* Below second standard deviation.
‡ Below first standard deviation.
§ Above first standard deviation.
‖ Above second standard deviation.
¶ X̄ Mean values of 40 healthy adults.
** 1S Values representing first standard deviation.
‡‡ 2S Values representing second standard deviation.

TABLE II

*Component Protein Concentration in C1r-Deficient and
Normal Human Serum*

Patient	C1q*	C1r‡	C1s§	C1s Inhibitor‖
	µg N/ml		*µg protein/ml*	*% of normal pool*
Brother	16	NB¶	11.7	280
Sister	20.8	NB	12.8	178
Normal	17–20	B**	30	100

* C1q was measured by the Mancini method of immunodiffusion using antisera prepared by the method of Morse and Christian (10).

‡ C1r was determined by the immunodiffusion method of Ouchterlony using prepared antisera according to the method of deBracco and Stroud (8). Quantitative determinations were not obtained at this stage.

§ C1s was measured by radial immunodiffusion according to the method of Nagaki and Stroud (16).

‖ C1s inhibitor was assayed by the Mancini method. The results are expressed as a percentage of the value in a normal serum pool.

¶ NB, no band.

** B, band.

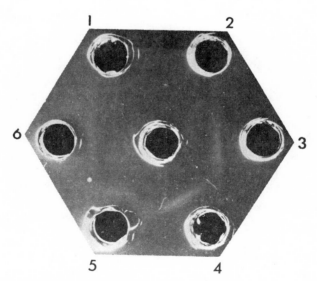

FIGURE 1 Immunodiffusion pattern by Ouchterlony of C1r-deficient patients using anti-C1r antiserum prepared against purified C1r. Well 1, undiluted serum from the brother; Well 2, undiluted serum from the sister; Well 3, normal serum; Well 4, C1 (kindly provided by R. Nelson); Well 5, normal serum diluted 1 : 2; Well 6, normal serum diluted 1 : 4.

99

Reconstitution of hemolytic C1 by purified C1r. To determine whether or not purified C1r would restore the hemolytic function, C1r was added to the patients' sera and incubated, and then C1 activity was assayed. The reconstitution experiments are based on the C1r assay method and use highly purified C1r as described by deBracco and Stroud (8). The assay cannot be done in whole serum if macromolecular C1 is detectable. In both the patients' sera, no C1 was detectable at a dilution of 1:100 after incubation for 45 min at 30°C (the specified

TABLE III
Reconstitution of C1 with Purified C1r

	Without C1r	C1r added
	units/ml	*units/ml*
Brother	0	2200
Sister	0	5000

Purified C1r, obtained as described (8), was added to 1:100 dilution of the patients' sera and incubated for 45 min at 30°C. C1 titers were then determined, but the EAC4 were washed before the addition of C2. C1r has no acitivity by itself in this assay, and is the limiting component. The units are C1 site forming units. C1r values were comparable to the values expected from the measured levels of C1q and C1s in the sister (see text).

time for C1r assays). It should be noted that after the serum dilutions were added to EAC4 and incubated, the cells were washed twice in low ionic strength-buffer solution but before C2 is added in order to remove free C1s. C1s alone has hemolytic activity (accounting for the routine C1 titers [Table I] in these patients), but it is not bound to EAC4 at low ionic strength. The fact that there are zero titers in the C1r assay indicates that all the activity is due to C1s and is not macromolecular C1.

As noted in Table III, significant activity could be restored in both sera. The amount of C1r activity added was also added to equivalent amounts of highly purified C1q and C1s, corresponding to the amount in the patients' serum. The titer in the female patient is essentially the same as found in these control mixtures. The regenerated activity was not as high in the patient with higher C1s inhibitor levels in spite of comparable C1s and C1q concentrations.

Bactericidal and immune adherence activity. Studies

of the bactericidal activity and immune adherence function of patients' sera deficient in Clr are presented in Table IV. The bactericidal activity against a rough strain of *E. coli* (Lilly) was markedly impaired as compared to normal in both the patients' sera. Immune adherence function was also reduced when the patients' sera were used with sensitized erythrocytes (EA). However, when sensitized cells carrying C1 EAC1 were used, immune adherence activity showed normal values, suggesting the inability of these sera to form EAC142.

Activation of the alternate pathway. Recently it has been emphasized that the complement system can be activated by alternate pathways (21-24). Sera deficient in Clr provided a useful new reagent with which to study the concept of the alternate pathways.

Table V represents data obtained when the patients sera and normal sera were treated with purified cobra venom factor, endotoxin, and immune complexes. As is shown in the table, no reduction in the concentration of Clq protein was demonstrable in either the CVF- or endotoxin-treated sera. Clq was utilized when antigen-antibody complexes were employed suggesting that the immunoglobulin binding site of Clq is functional and occurs in the absence of Clr.

The utilization of C4 and C2 with CVF was less than 10% (Table V). However, the consumption of C3 was approximately 90%. To a variable degree consumption of terminal components other than C3 was observed with the patients' sera and cobra venom factor. When endotoxin was used (Table V) minimal consumption of earlier components in both normal and patients sera occurred. By contrast, regular consumption of large amounts of C3 was observed. Finally, regular consumption of the later components C5–C9 was somewhat variable in degree. When antigen-antibody complexes were used to activate the complement system, minimal utilization of C4 was seen with both of the patients sera. C2 and to a greater extent C3, C6, and C7 were fixed by the brother's serum suggesting that the brother's later components can be activated by antigen-antibody complexes to some extent without the utilization of earlier components.

DISCUSSION

In this report we have analyzed in detail the complement system in all the surviving members of a family in which deficiency of Clr is associated with serious clinical disease. In the affected brother a gross deficiency or absence of hemolytic C1 and of C1r was associated with skin, renal and joint disease, and vasculitis clinically suggestive of lupus erythematosus. In the second patient the deficiency of C1r was associated with frequent infections, arthralgia, and recurrent skin lesions. Although

TABLE IV

Bactericidal Activity and Immune Adherence Function of Sera Deficient in C1r

	Bactericidal activity*	Immune	adherence‡
Patient	*E. coli*§	EA‖	EAC1 ¶
Brother	0.048	10	160
Sister	0.081	10	160
Normal	0.0072	320	320

* Bactericidal activity performed according to the method of Muschel and Treffers (20). Results are expressed as the amount of serum necessary to kill 50% of bacteria.
‡ Immune adherence function according to the method of Nishioka (19). Results are expressed as the reciprocal of dilutions of serum.
§ Rough strain *E. coli* (Lilly).
‖ Sheep erythrocytes sensitized with rabbit antibody.
¶ Sensitized sheep erythrocytes containing C1.

three living siblings are normal and have been found to have hemolytically normal C1, the family history revealed that another male died in late childhood of a lupus-like syndrome similar to that of his living affected brother. Further, two siblings died in infancy probably from infection. The father and mother have normal levels of hemolytic C1. Using monospecific antiserum, C1r could not be detected in the serum of the two children even by highly sensitive Ouchterlony and radial immunodiffusion assays. It seems likely from this family study that we are dealing with a genetically determined inborn error of metabolism. Although the precise nature of the genetic fault can be established only by a more complete quantitative analysis of the C1r concentrations and by a more complete genetic analysis, the occurrence of the defect and associated serious disease in several male and female siblings of apparently healthy parents who have several healthy offspring suggests an autosomal recessive inheritance. Hemolytic C1 as titrated by this method may be normal even though a heterozygous state with partial deficiency of C1r is present. The coexistence of

C1r deficiency and renal disease has previously been described by Pickering, Naff, Stroud, Good, and Gewurz (4). Thus it seems more than coincidental that serious renal-vascular disease is associated with a defect of the C1r component of the complement system. Moreover, the study in this family suggests that the error is congenital and not acquired. In the patient of Pickering et al. perturbations of the complement system in addition to the deficiency of C1 were noticed. A decreased concentration of C1s was present, C4 was elevated, and an increase in C1 esterase inhibitor was also recorded. In both of our C1r deficient patients these same perturbations of the complement system were found. The significance of the elevation of both the hemolytic C4 and C1-esterase inhibitor is not clear but C4 is a substrate for C1s and C1r may be important in the activation of C1s (25). Thus, in the absence of C1r, C4 may be protected from destruction or utilization. The C1s inhibitor fluctuates with several disease states for unknown reasons and may represent a compensatory mechanism in chronic inflammation (26). Alternatively this component may behave as an acute phase reactant. We have no proven explanation for the consistently low levels of C1s in these patients.

Deficient hemolytic activity of the complement system attributable to a defect of C1 was reported by Pondman, Stoop, Cormane, and Hannema (5), This defect correctable by addition of purified C1s was also associated with a lupus-like syndrome. In our patients, on the other hand, hemolytic activity was restored in both patients by addition of purified C1r to the serum. Quantitatively when equal amounts of C1r were added the restoration was greater in the male than in the female patient. The difference in restoration provided by C1r in this experiment is probably attributable to differences in the concentration of the C1-esterase inhibitor. The effected sister had higher concentration of the inhibitor than did the male patient. Ratnoff, Pensky, Ogston, and Naff (27) have previously shown that this inhibitor blocks the activity of C1r as well as that of C1-esterase.

Of further interest is the observation that levels of all of the terminal complement components C3–C9 were elevated in the serum of the male patient while some of the terminal components C3, C5, and C9 were elevated in the serum of his sister. Although the significance of these increases must await further analysis it is provocative that our family study revealed that the healthy family members all showed high total serum complement hemolytic activity, increases of some of the later com-

TABLE V

Alternate Pathways of The C System in C1r-Deficient Sera

	Immunodiffusion* C1q‡ (µg N/ml)	% Consumption								
		C1	C4	C2	C3	C5	C6	C7	C8	C9
Brother+CVF§	7.8	—	<10	<10	88	31	25	<10	<10	17
Sister+CVF	8.6	—	<10	<10	90	30	45	38	30	<10
Normal+CVF	8.2	<10	<10	<10	88	25	21	<10	33	<10
Brother+Endotoxin‖	11.2	—	26	35	85	26	33	42	45	25
Sister+Endotoxin	12.9	—	18	22	80	34	45	45	35	22
Normal+Endotoxin	9.2	<10	24	22	90	28	27	17	31	55
Brother+AgAb¶	2.4	—	15	16	56	13	39	44	<10	<10
Sister+AgAb	1.4	—	25	<10	17	21	12	<10	<10	15
Normal+AgAb	0.6	>90	>90	>90	>90	46	32	42	15	30

The results are expressed as the per cent inhibition of normal saline controls.
* Immunodiffusion was carried out according to the method of Mancini (15).
‡ Measurement of C1q was done with antisera prepared according to the method of Morse & Christian (10).
§ Purified cobra venom factor.
‖ Endotoxin E. coli (Lilly).
¶ Immune complex (BSA rabbit anti-BSA), CVF (2 µg/ml), endotoxin (15 mg/ml), and Ag-Ab (2 mg/ml) were interacted with equal volumes of serum, respectively, and incubated at 37°C for 30 min before testing. Controls consisted of respective reactants and saline.

ponents, and consistent elevations of C8. Perhaps further genetic analysis will reveal the meaning of these associations. Little is known of the basis for increases in terminal complement component concentrations, but elevations of total complement and complement components on a familial basis might reflect increased stimulation by the more frequent infections which feature the clinical disease. Further studies of the family from this point of view seem desirable.

We found further that using bacterial endotoxin and cobra venom, activators of the alternative pathways (22-24, 28, 29), the complement system could be engaged in the absence of C1r. The absence of C1r did not completely prevent activation of the complement system even by antigen-antibody complexes. Of the later components especially C3, C6, and C7 were utilized upon activation of the system with Ag-Ab complexes. This observation supports the finding of Sandberg, Osler, Shin, and Oliveira (21) that Fab₂ fragments can engage an alternate pathway into the complement system. It is remotely possible that very small amounts of C1r undetectable by the sensitive methods used in this study are sufficient to permit some activation of the C system by the conventional pathway and it is difficult to be certain that serum preparations are completely free of endotoxin. However, both saline controls and BSA controls failed to show activation of the terminal components of the C system in these sera. Surprisingly the sera of the two C1r-deficient siblings behaved differently in the experiment in which Ag-Ab complexes were used to activate the C system. In the male patient clear evidence of activation of the terminal components was observed while in the female relatively little evidence for activation was found. Perhaps the difference may be due to a more efficient alternative pathway in the male than in the female. Both sera on the other hand permitted activation of terminal components with endotoxin and CVF.

Studies of the C1r-deficient serum showed deficient bactericidal activity as well as deficiencies in development of immune adherence and facilitation of phagocytosis.[3] The deficiency in bactericidal activity was to be anticipated since Goldman, Ruddy, Austen, and Feingold

---

[3] Biggar, W. D., N. K. B. Day, D. Windhorst, and R. A. Good. Impaired phagocytosis in C1r-deficient sera. Submitted for publication.

have previously shown that intact C1 is essential for bactericidal function (30).

The central question posed by the study of our patients with C1r deficiency as well as of the patient studied by Pickering et al. (4) is: How does the isolated absence of C1r predispose to the associated clinical and pathological disorders that have been observed? Perhaps the deficiency of C1r favors selective use of alternative pathways into the complement system, that are more likely to be associated with destructive inflammatory or vascular reactivity than is the conventional pathway utilizing the intact first component of the complement cascade. It could be that the deficiency of C1r and C1r-dependent actions of the complement system increases susceptibility to infection, as was especially clear in the clinical history of the sister, and that this in some way leads to the vasculitis. Utilization of active C1s has not been ruled out but high levels of C4 and normal levels of C2 are against this possibility. The medical history of the several siblings in this family, indicating that the absence of C1r is associated with an increased frequency of infection, suggests the possibility that C1r or the intact complement cascade has a major function in host defense and that the absence of this component causes a susceptibility to infection with microorganisms capable of producing the lesions observed.

ACKNOWLEDGMENTS

We wish to thank Mrs. Linda Campbell and Mrs. Linda Schuveiller for their excellent technical assistance.

This work was aided by a grant from the U. S. Public Health Service (AI-08677), The National Foundation-March of Dimes, the American Heart Association, and the Arthritis Foundation.

REFERENCES

1. Gewurz, H., R. J. Pickering, C. L. Christian, R. Snyderman, S. E. Mergenhagen, and R. A. Good. 1968. Decreased C1q protein concentration and agglutinating activity in agammaglobulinemia syndromes: an inborn error reflected in the complement system. *Clin. Exp. Immunol.* 3: 437.
2. Gewurz, H., R. J. Pickering, and R. A. Good. 1968. Complement and complement component activities in diseases associated with repeated infections and malignancy. *Int. Arch. Allergy Appl. Immunol.* 33: 368.
3. Kohler, P. F., and H. J. Müller-Eberhard. 1969. Complement-immunoglobulin relation: deficiency of C1q associated with impaired IgG synthesis. *Science (Washington).* 163: 474.

4. Pickering, R. J., G. B. Naff, R. M. Stroud, R. A. Good, and H. Gewurz. 1970. Deficiency of C1r in human serum. Effects of the structure and function of macromolecular C1. *J. Exp. Med.* **141**: 803.

5. Pondman, K. W., J. W. Stoop, R. H. Cormane, and A. J. Hannema. 1968. Abnormal C1 in a patient with systemic lupus erythematosus. *J. Immunol.* **101**: 811.

6. Mayer, M. M. 1961. Procedure for titration of complement. *In* Experimental Immunochemistry. E. A. Kabat M. M. Mayer, editors. Charles C Thomas, Publisher, Springfield, Ill. 163.

7. Yonemasu, K., and J. Stroud. 1971. C1q: rapid purification method for preparation of monospecific antiserum and for biochemical studies. *J. Immunol.* **106**: 304.

8. Debracco, M. M. E., and R. M. Stroud. 1971. C1r, subunit of the first C component; purification, properties and assay based on its linking role. *J. Clin. Invest.* **50**: 838.

9. Nagaki, K., and R. M. Stroud. 1970. A method for preparing monospecific antiserum to C1 esterase. *J. Immunol.* **105**: 162.

10. Morse, J. H., and C. L. Christian. 1964. Immunological studies of the 11S protein component of the human complement system. *J. Exp. Med.* **119**: 195.

11. Nelson, R. A., Jr., J. Jensen, I. Gigli, and N. Tamura. 1966. Methods for the separation, purification and measurement of nine components of hemolytic complement in guinea pig serum. *Immunochemistry.* **3**: 111.

12. Gewurz, H., A. R. Page, R. J. Pickering, and R. A. Good. 1967. Complement activity and neutrophil exudation in man. Studies in patients with glomerulonephritis, essential hypocomplementemia and agammaglobulinemia. *Int. Arch. Allergy Appl. Immunol.* **32**: 64.

13. Borsos, T., and H. Rapp. 1967. Immune hemolysis: a simplified method for the preparation of EAC4 with guinea pig or with human complement. *J. Immunol.* **99**: 263.

14. Day, N. K. B., R. J. Pickering, H. Gewurz, and R. A. Good. 1969. Ontogenetic development of the complement system. *Immunology.* **16**: 319.

15. Mancini, J., A. O. Carbonara, and J. F. Heremans. 1965. Immunochemical quantitation of antigens by single radial immunodiffusion. *Immunochemistry.* **2**: 235.

16. Nagaki, K., and R. M. Stroud. 1970. A method for preparing monospecific antiserum to C1 esterase. *J. Immunol.* **105**: 162.

17. Nelson, R. A. 1966. A new concept of immunosuppression in hypersensitivity reactions and in transplantation immunity. *Surv. Ophthalmol.* **11**: 498.

18. Day, N. K. B., H. Gewurz, R. Johannsen, J. Finstad, and R. A. Good. 1970. Complement and complement like activity in lower vertebrates and invertebrates. *J. Exp. Med.* **132**: 941.

19. Nishioka, K. 1963. Measurement of complement agglutination of human erythrocytes reacting in immune adherence. *J. Immunol.* **90**: 86.

20. Muschel, L. H., and H. B. Treffers. 1956. Quantitative

studies on the bactericidal actions of serum and of complement. *J. Immunol.* **76**: 1.

21. Sandberg, A. L., A. G. Osler, H. S. Shin, and B. Oliveira. 1970. The biologic activities of guinea pig antibodies: modes of complement interaction with gamma 1 and gamma 2 immunoglobulins. *J. Immunol.* **104**: 329.

22. Götze, O., and H. J. Müller-Eberhard. 1971. The C3-activator system: an alternate pathway of C activition. *J. Exp. Med.* **134** (Suppl. I) : 96.

23. Marcus, R. L., H. S. Shin, and M. Mayer. 1971. An alternate complement pathway: C3-cleaving activity not due to C4,2a on endotoxic lipopolysaccharide after treatment with guinea pig serum. Relation to properdin. *Proc. Nat. Acad. Sci.* **68**: 1351.

24. Frank, M. M., J. May, T. Gaither, and E. Ellman. 1971. In vitro studies of C function in sera of C4-deficient guinea pigs. *J. Exp. Med.* **134**: 178.

25. Naff, G. B., and O. D. Ratnoff. 1968. The enzymatic nature of C1r. *J. Exp. Med.* **128**: 571.

26. Donaldson, V. H. 1966. Serum inhibitor of C1 esterase in health and disease. *J. Lab. Clin. Med.* **68**: 369.

27. Ratnoff, O. D., J. Pensky, D. Ogston, and G. B. Naff. 1969. The inhibition of plasmin, plasma kallikrein, plasma permeability factor and C1r subcomponent of the first component of complement by serum C1 esterase inhibitor. *J. Exp. Med.* **129**: 515.

28. Gewurz, H., H. S. Shin, and S. E. Mergenhagen. 1968. Interactions of the complement system with endotoxic lipopolysaccharide. Consumption of each of the six terminal complement components. *J. Exp. Med.* **128**: 1049.

29. Gewurz, H. 1971. Alternate pathways to damage of membranes to complement. Proceedings of the International Symposium on the Biological Activities of Complement. D. G. Ingram, editor. S. Karger, Basel. In press.

30. Goldman, J. N., S. Ruddy, K. F. Austen, and D. S. Feingold. 1969. The serum bactericidal reaction. III. Antibody and complement requirements for killing a rough *Escherichia coli*. *J. Immunol.* **102**: 1378.

The relation of type of initial symptoms and line of transmission to ages at onset and death in Huntington's disease

C. J. BRACKENRIDGE

The considerable variation in the natural history and phenomenology of Huntington's disease has long been recognized. Davenport & Muncey (1916) coined the term 'biotype' to express the similarity of the clinical picture within some families and the differences occurring among families. "Thus there is a biotype in which tremors are absent, but mental deterioration present; a biotype in which the tremors are not accompanied by mental deterioration; a biotype in which the chorea does not progress; and a biotype in which the onset of the choreic movements is in early life."

Over the ensuing years the heterogeneity has largely simplified into three or four variants; the classical, juvenile, and Westphal types have been discussed by Bruyn (1968), who also refers to a minor type termed 'status subchoreaticus' by Patzig (1935). Burch (1968) has proposed that predisposition to Huntington's disease is determined by a single autosomal gene with dominant effect and that its particular form depends upon one or more modifying genes at one or more other loci.

Clinical descriptions in the literature seldom permit unequivocal classification of cases into one of these variants. In the present study the approach adopted, which recalls the nosology of Meierhofer (1937), was to group subjects according to whether

This work was supported by a grant from the National Health and Medical Research Council of Australia.

neurological or psychiatric symptoms appeared first or whether they coincided. Two neurological signs were distinguished (A) choreo-athetosis, usually associated with hyperkinesia, hallmarks of the classical variant and (B) muscular rigidity, usually associated with hypokinesia, hallmarks of the Westphal variant. The aim was to determine whether the ages at onset and at death were related to the early symptomatology of the disorder.

Material and Method

Sibship records derived *seriatim* from published case reports and pedigrees were subjected to two preliminary selection tests:

(A) Unless all members of a sibship were affected with Huntington's disease, only sibships succeeded by at least two generations of offspring of direct or indirect descent at the time of ascertainment were included in the material for analysis. This was designed to ensure that cases of late onset were not omitted.

(B) If the sex of the affected parent could not be determined with certainty, the sibship was excluded from analysis. In this way any non-hereditary forms of chorea were discarded.

Of the 1,561 sibships initially assembled, 878 (56.2 %) remained after applying these constraints. These were then scrutinized for information regarding the type of symptoms at the onset of illness. Subjects were divided into three clinical groups according to whether neurological signs preceded psychiatric symptoms, neurological signs were essentially coincident with psychiatric symptoms, or neurological signs followed psychiatric symptoms. The number of sibships with one or more members so classified was 201 (12.9 % of those initially assembled). The greatest single contribution was 27 sibships described by Muncey (1964).

Data on type of neurological signs (chorea-hyperkinesia or rigidity-hypokinesia), sex, age at onset, age at death, duration of illness of affected subjects, and sexes of affected parents and grandparents were recorded when available. No attempt was made to group subjects according to type of psychiatric disorder because of the large number and wide range of overlapping states involved: these included antisocial behaviour; character changes; affective, personality, and psychotic disorders; and organic dementia. The Appendix summarizes some clinical details and sources of the subjects.

The data were processed for a Fortran program (MANOVA) of the University of Miami Biometric Laboratory for multivariate analyses of variance involving five factors (clinical group, type of neurological sign, sex of subject, sex of affected parent, and sex of affected grandparent) and three variables (age at onset, age at death, and duration of illness).

Results and Discussion

To determine whether the distributions of affected subjects according to sex and clinical group differed appreciably from equal proportions, the values in the Appendix were analysed. Of 292 subjects, 144 were males and 148 were females; the sex ratio is clearly close to unity. This result contrasts with the preponderance of affected males found previously in a fourfold larger sample of cases unselected for type of initial symptoms (Brackenridge 1971). The reason for this difference is unknown.

With regard to type of symptoms, 114 (39.0 %) first presented with neurological signs, 84 (28.8 %) first presented with psychiatric symptoms, and in 94 (32.2 %) their onset could not be separated. Oepen, Landzettel, Streletzki & von Koppenfels (1963) reported that in 219 cases, symptoms at onset were primarily motor in 74 (33.8 %), behavioural in 53 (24.2 %), and simultaneous in 92 (42.0 %). Brothers (1964) recorded different proportions in his ascertainment of cases in Victoria, Australia. Of 237 subjects, the first symptoms were chorea in 140 (59.1 %), personality and character change in 66 (27.8 %), and in 31 (13.1 %) it was impossible to state accurately which appeared first. The frequencies of Oepen et al. (1963) and the present series do not differ significantly ($G = 5.21$ for 2 d.f., $P > 0.05$) whereas the frequencies of Brothers (1964) are significantly different from those of Oepen et al. (1963) ($G = 53.04$, $P < 0.001$) and from those of the present study ($G = 32.36$, $P < 0.001$). It is possible that the proportions of each type of symptom vary with geographical location, in which case more documentation will be necessary before the suggestion can be properly tested.

Fathers exceeded mothers as the affected parent of subjects in each clinical group (Table 1). The total sex ratio of 167/125 (1.34) differs significantly from unity due largely to the contribution of subjects who displayed neurological and psychiatric symptoms simultaneously. Attention has been drawn on several occasions to the predominance of transmitting fathers in cases of early onset (Bruyn 1968, Merrit, Conneally, Rahman & Drew 1969). It is therefore possible that the present excess arose from the number of juvenile patients in the sample. To test this hypothesis, the analysis was repeated on affected parents of offspring presenting with symptoms before and after the age of 20 years. In the former group, the parental sex ratio of 37/12 (3.08) was significantly higher ($G = 7.83$, $P < 0.01$) than in the latter group which had a ratio of 107/96 (1.11). The suggestion is therefore supported by these results. (It is to be noted that the parental figures so far quoted are partly artificial. They refer to parents of siblings and not to parents of sibships; because sibships may contain more than one affected sibling, a given parent may have been counted more than once. This is unavoidable since the type of clinical symptoms and quantitative variables such as onset age may vary appreciably within a sibship.) The main finding of a paternal preponderance is sustained when affected parental sex is determined for all sibships, the ratio of 119/82 (1.45) being significantly higher than unity ($G = 6.48$, $P < 0.02$).

The distribution in Table 1 of the four parental-grandparental lines of transmission among the three clinical groups is significantly heterogeneous ($G = 15.18$ for 6 d.f., $P < 0.02$). For the whole sample the proportions differ significantly from 1:1:1:1 owing to the contributions of subjects in whom motor signs preceded or accompanied psychiatric symptoms. Only when the latter foreshadowed neurological signs did the father-grandfather and mother-grandfather lines fail to exceed the other lines of descent. An interesting feature of the distribution is that subjects from parental-grandparental lines of the same sex are similar in number to those from lines of different sex, regardless of the clinical group to which they belong. The excess of cases arising from the paternal grandfather has been noted previously (Haldane 1941, Brackenridge 1971). In the light of the present results it seems that the precise proportions of each line of transmission will depend on the proportions of subjects in the three clinical groups. The reason for the effect is elusive but as the area of applicability becomes more clearly defined, its basis may be revealed. The distributions of the four lines of descent showed no significant heterogeneity when choreic and rigid patients were compared.

In Table 2 the age at onset, age at death, and duration of symptoms are expressed as functions of the type of clinical presentation and neurological signs of the subjects. The most striking features of the results are the

Table 1

Distribution of subjects of three clinical groups according to sex of affected parent and line of transmission

Clinical group	Affected parent		Test of goodnes of fit to equal proportions		Line of transmission				Test of goodness of fit to equal proportions	
	Father	Mother	G	P	Father-grand-father	Father-grand-mother	Mother-grand-father	Mother-grand-mother	G	P
Neurological signs before psychiatric symptoms	62	52	0.88	> 0.3	36	17	25	11	15.83	< 0.005
Neurological signs coincident with psychiatric symptoms	58	36	5.20	< 0.025	32	12	23	6	23.17	< 0.001
Neurological signs after psychiatric symptoms	47	37	1.19	> 0.2	11	16	18	14	1.86	> 0.5
Total	167	125	6.06	< 0.02	79	45	66	31	25.67	< 0.001

Table 2

Age at onset, age at death, and duration of illness in years of affected subjects according to clinical group and neurological sign

Clinical group	Neurological sign	Age at onset			Age at death			Duration of illness		
		Mean	S.E.	No.	Mean	S.E.	No.	Mean	95 % limits*	No.
Neurological signs before psychiatric symptoms	Chorea	38.73	1.24	77	56.17	1.53	72	13.01	10.94-15.48	50
	Rigidity	28.56	6.55	9	40.00	7.34	9	9.80	4.94-19.46	8
Neurological signs coincident with psychiatric symptoms	Chorea	36.17	1.40	66	46.14	1.92	36	9.02	7.15-11.38	35
	Rigidity	18.00	2.44	26	25.86	3.69	14	8.23	6.15-11.02	14
Neurological signs after psychiatric symptoms	Chorea	32.91	1.60	56	48.58	1.83	33	14.48	11.57-18.12	30
	Rigidity	24.06	3.09	18	39.73	4.33	11	12.73	10.50-15.43	11

* 95 % fiducial limits replace the S.E. because duration of illness is logarithmically distributed.

decreased values associated with rigidity when compared with choreiform movements. Analyses of variance of age at onset, age at death, and duration of illness were therefore performed; the factors to be tested for significance being clinical group, neurological sign, sex of subject, sex of affected parent, and sex of affected grandparent.

Table 3 demonstrates that clinical picture, neurological sign, and sex of subject and affected parent are all significant determinants of age at onset of symptoms. The strong interaction between clinical group and neurological sign reflects the significant heterogeneity (G = 13.69 for 2 d.f., P < 0.005) in the extent of rigidity in the three groups, the frequency being greatest when abnormal behaviour and spasticity appear together (Table 2). The strong interaction between neurological sign and sex of subject is also of interest. Examination of the whole sample shows that of 238 choreic subjects, 110 were males and 128 were females whereas of 54 rigid-hypokinetic subjects, 34 were

males and 20 were females. The heterogeneity is significant (G = 4.32, P < 0.05).

The variation of onset age with type of first symptoms may reflect topographical differences in the site of attack. Oepen *et. al.* (1963) found, in agreement with the results of Table 2, that age at onset was earliest when initial symptoms were psychiatric in character but their observed differences were not significant. The present finding that rigidity-hypokinesia is associated with a lower onset age than classical choreic symptoms is consistent with the report that the mean onset age in subjects with the Westphal variant is 22 years (Bittenbender & Quadfasel 1962).

The observation that both sex of subject and sex of affected parent are related to age at first symptoms is surprising in view of the previous failure to find any significant differences (Brackenridge 1971). The reason may be that rigidity is over-represented in the present study because Westphal cases are of exceptional interest and clinical data are more likely to be available

Table 3

Analysis of variance of age at onset

Source	d.f.	Mean square	F	P <
Main effects				
Clinical group	2	1003.249	7.865	0.001
Neurological sign	1	3869.811	30.339	0.001
Sex of subject	1	631.714	4.953	0.028
Sex of affected parent	1	524.613	4.113	0.044
Sex of affected grandparent	1	46.234	0.362	0.548
First order interactions				
Clinical group-neurological sign	2	479.995	3.763	0.025
Clinical group-sex of subject	2	149.414	1.171	0.313
Clinical group-sex of affected parent	2	10.053	0.079	0.924
Clinical group-sex of affected grandparent	2	142.758	1.119	0.329
Neurological sign-sex of subject	1	699.863	5.487	0.020
Neurological sign-sex of affected parent	1	349.743	2.742	0.100
Neurological sign-sex of affected grandparent	1	88.277	0.692	0.407
Sex of subject-sex of affected parent	1	15.955	0.125	0.724
Sex of subject-sex of affected grandparent	1	44.917	0.352	0.554
Sex of affected parent-sex of affected grandparent	1	153.924	1.207	0.274
Higher order interactions	19	136.572	1.071	0.387
Within cells	150	127.554		

for them than for typical cases. The previously described difference in sex ratio between choreic and rigid subjects and the fact that fathers exceed mothers as affected parents to a significantly greater extent $(G = 7.18, P < 0.01)$ for rigid-akinetic patients (40/14) than for classical choreic patients (127/111) may then explain the observation.

Table 4 demonstrates that age at death

Table 4

Analysis of variance of age at death

Source	d.f.	Mean square	F	P <
Main effects				
Clinical group	2	2835.176	17.703	0.001
Neurological sign	1	3629.408	22.662	0.001
Sex of subject	1	1269.015	7.924	0.006
Sex of affected parent	1	991.387	6.190	0.015
Sex of affected grandparent	1	0.726	0.005	0.946
First-order interactions				
Clinical group-neurological sign	2	233.886	1.460	0.238
Clinical group-sex of subject	2	134.952	0.843	0.434
Clinical group-sex of affected parent	2	62.740	0.392	0.677
Clinical group-sex of affected grandparent	2	36.559	0.228	0.796
Neurological sign-sex of subject	1	475.560	2.969	0.088
Neurological sign-sex of affected parent	1	473.886	2.959	0.089
Neurological sign-sex of affected grandparent	1	342.385	2.138	0.147
Sex of subject-sex of affected parent	1	20.223	0.126	0.723
Sex of subject-sex of affected grandparent	1	20.991	0.131	0.718
Sex of affected parent-sex of affected grandparent	1	19.292	0.120	0.720
Higher order interactions	17	190.005	1.186	0.291
Within cells	91	160.155		

Table 5

Analysis of variance of duration of illness (logarithmically transformed)

Source	d.f.	Mean square	F	P <
Main effects				
Clinical group	2	2.012	5.878	0.004
Neurological sign	1	0.533	1.556	0.216
Sex of subject	1	0.028	0.081	0.777
Sex of affected parent	1	1.131	3.305	0.073
Sex of affected grandparent	1	0.055	0.161	0.689
First-order interactions				
Clinical group-neurological sign	2	0.167	0.488	0.616
Clinical group-sex of subject	2	0.074	0.216	0.806
Clinical group-sex of affected parent	2	0.072	0.210	0.811
Clinical group-sex of affected grandparent	2	1.927	5.629	0.005
Neurological sign-sex of subject	1	0.443	1.295	0.259
Neurological sign-sex of affected parent	1	0.230	0.672	0.415
Neurological sign-sex of affected grandparent	1	0.006	0.017	0.896
Sex of subject-sex of affected parent	1	0.057	0.166	0.685
Sex of subject-sex of affected grandparent	1	0.452	1.320	0.254
Sex of affected parent-sex of affected grandparent	1	0.048	0.141	0.708
Higher order interactions	17	0.468	1.368	0.180
Within cells	70	0.342		

is strongly affected by the same factors as age at onset without any of the interactions reaching a significant level of probability. On the other hand, the duration of illness is determined only by the early clinical manifestations (Table 5). The unexpected interaction between clinical group and sex of affected grandparent is difficult to explain in view of its absence from Tables 3 and 4. Examination of the whole sample shows that affected grandparental sex displays a significantly heterogeneous distribution among the clinical groups (G = 10.39 for 2 d.f., P < 0.01). Apparently this relationship is not disturbed by the interactions between duration and grandparental sex and between duration and clinical group whereas it is disturbed in the analyses reported in Tables 3 and 4.

The strong effects of early clinical symptoms, neurological signs, sex of subject, and sex of affected parent upon ages at onset and at death call for further studies to determine their clinical and genetic bases. One approach being examined is to attempt discrimination of the material into discrete populations which may lead to a clarification of the mechanisms responsible.

References

Althaus, J. (1880). Chorea mit Epilepsie gepaart. *Arch. Psychiat. Nervenkr.* **10**, 139–145.

Arai, Y., A. Goto, T. Majima, K. Murofushi & H. Narabayashi (1968). Two cases of Huntington's chorea. Clinical and neuropathological studies of a typical and an atypical form in a family. *Clin. Neurol. (Tokyo)* **8**, 635–642.

Baron, G. (1950). Contribution à l'étude clinique et génétique des chorées chroniques progressives familiales maladie de Huntington et états Huntingtonniers. Thesis, Faculté de Médecine de Paris.

Beaubrun, M. H. (1963). Huntington's chorea in Trinidad. *W. Indian med. J.* **12**, 39–46.

Becker, G. (1938). Beitrag zur Klinik und Genealogie der Huntingtonschen Chorea. *Allg. Z. Psychiat.* **107**, 193–232.

Bell, J. (1934). Nervous disease and muscular dystrophies. Part I. Huntington's chorea. *The Treasury of Human Inheritance,* ed. R. A. Fisher & L. S. Penrose. Cambridge University Press, London.

Bittenbender, J. B. & F. A. Quadfasel (1962). Rigid and akinetic forms of Huntington's chorea. *Arch. Neurol. (Chic.)* **7**, 275–288.

Brackenridge, C. J. (1971). A genetic and statistical study of some sex-related factors in Huntington's disease. *Clin. Genet.* **2**, 267-286.

Briebrecher, G. (1938). C..orea Huntington-Sippe. Dissertation, University of Bonn.

Brothers, C. R. D. (1964). Huntington's chorea in Victoria and Tasmania, *J. neurol. Sci.* **1**, 405–420.

Brothers, C. R. D. & A. W. Meadows (1955). An investigation of Huntington's chorea in Victoria. *J. ment. Sci.* **101**, 548–563.

Bruyn, G. W. (1968). Huntington's chorea. Historical, clinical and laboratory synopsis. *Handbook of Clinical Neurology,* ed. P. J. Vinken & G. W. Bruyn, Vol. 6, pp. 298–378. North-Holland, Amsterdam.

Buck, C. A. (1934). Huntington's chorea, with the report of a case. *Canad. med. Ass. J.* **31**, 178–180.

Burch, P. R. J. (1968). Huntington's chorea. Age at onset in relation to aetiology and pathogenesis. *Handbook of Clinical Neurology,* ed. P. J. Vinken & G. W. Bruyn, Vol. 6, pp. 379–398. North-Holland, Amsterdam.

Byers, R. K. & J. A. Dodge (1967). Huntington's chorea in children. Report of four cases. *Neurology (Minneap.)* **17**, 587–596.

Campbell, A. M. G., B. Corner, R. M. Norman & H. Urich (1961). The rigid form of Huntington's disease. *J. Neurol. Neurosurg. Psychiat.* **24**, 71–77.

Chhuttani, P. N. (1955). Huntington's chorea in the Punjab (India). *J. Ass. Phycns India* **3**, 40–45.

Curran, D. (1930). Huntington's chorea without choreiform movements. *J. Neurol. Psychopath.* **10**, 305–310.

Curschmann, H. (1908). Eine neue Chorea-Huntingtonfamilie. *Dtsch. Z. Nervenheilk.* **35**, 293–305.

Davenport, C. B. & Muncey, E. B. (1916). Huntington's chorea in relation to heredity and eugenics. *Amer. J. Insan.* **73**, 195–222.

Delmas-Marsalet, P., M. Bourgeois, C. Vital & X. Fontanges (1968). Formes rigides de la maladie de Huntington (étude d'une famille avec un cas anatomo-clinique). *Rev. neurol.* **118**, 273–283.

De Marco, P. & G. Testa (1969). La forma infanto-prepuberale della corea di Huntington. *G. Psichiat. Neuropat.* **3**, 391–403.

Dewhurst, K. (1970). Personality disorder in Huntington's disease. *Psychiat. clin.* **3**, 221–229.

Dewhurst, K. & J. Oliver (1970). Huntington's disease of young people. *Europ. Neurol.* **3**, 278–289.

D'Ormea, A. (1904). Una famiglia coreica. *Rif. med.* **20**, 313–318.

Entres, J. L. (1921). Zur Klinik und Vererbung der Huntington'schen Chorea. *Monographien aus dem Gesamtgebiet der Neurologie u. Psychiatrie*, Heft 37. Springer-Verlag, Berlin.

Evans, J. J. W. (1908). Observations on a case of Huntington's chorea. *Lancet* **2**, 940.

Frank, W. (1937). Untersuchungen über Chorea Huntington an Hand von 19 Fällen unter besonderer Berucksichtigung der Erblichkeit und der Fruhsymptome, *Psychiat.-neurol. Wschr.* **39**, 51–58.

Frets, G. P. (1943). De erfelijkheid bij 15 lijders aan chronische, progressieve chorea (Huntington), die in de jaren 1914–1941 in de psychiatrische inrichting "Maasoord" verpleegd zijn. *Genetica* **23**, 465–528.

Gaule, A. (1932). Das Auftreten der Chorea Huntington in einer Familie der Nordostschweiz. *Schweiz Arch. Neurol. Psychiat.* **29**, 90–112.

Geratovitsch, M. (1927). Über Erblichkeitsuntersuchungen bei der Huntington'schen Krankheit. *Arch. Psychiat. Nervenkr.* **80**, 513–535.

Gezelle Meerburg, G. F. (1923). Bijdrage naar aanleiding van een anatomisch en genealogisch onderzoek tot de kennis van de chorea Huntingtonea. Thesis, University of Utrecht.

Goldstein, M. (1913). Ein kasuistischer Beitrag zur Chorea chronica hereditaria. *Münch. med. Wschr.* **60**, 1659–1662.

Goodman, R. M., C. L. Hall, L. Terango, G. A. Perrine & P. L. Roberts (1966). Huntington's chorea: a multidisciplinary study of affected parents and first generation offspring. *Arch. Neurol. (Chic.)* **15**, 345–355.

Gröpl, H. (1968). Chorea Huntington im Kindesalter. *Z. Kinderheilk.* **103**, 45–51.

Haldane, J. B. S. (1941). The relative importance of principal and modifying genes in determining some human diseases. *J. Genet.* **41**, 149–157.

Hamilton, A. S. (1908). A report of twenty-seven cases of chronic progressive chorea. *Amer. J. Insan.* **64**, 403–475.

Hempel, H. C. (1938). Ein Beitrag zur Huntingtonschen Erkrankung. *Z. ges. Neurol. Psychiat.* **160**, 563–597.

Hoffmann, J. (1888). Ueber Chorea chronica progressiva (Huntington'sche Chorea, Chorea hereditaria). *Virchows Arch. path. Anat.* **111**, 513–548.

Huber, A. (1887). Chorea hereditaria der Erwachsenen (Huntington'sche Chorea). *Virchows Arch. path. Anat.* **108**, 267–285.

Huet, E. (1889). De la chorée chronique. Thesis, University of Paris.

Jervis, G. A. (1963). Huntington's chorea in childhood. *Arch. Neurol. (Chic.)* **9**, 244–257.

Kalkhof, J. & O. Ranke (1913). Eine neue Chorea Huntington-Familie. *Z. ges. Neurol. Psychiat.* **17**, 256–302.

Kloos, G. (1938). Gehaufte erbliche Taubheit in einer Huntington-Familie. *Münch. med. Wschr.* **85**, 94–96.

Lannois, M. (1888). Chorée hereditaire. *Rev. Méd. (Paris)* **8**, 645–681.

Leese, S. M., D. A. Pond & J. Shields (1952). A pedigree of Huntington's chorea. *Ann. Eugen. (Lond.)* **17**, 92–112.

Mackenzie-van der Noordaa, M. C. (1960). De door Westphal beschreven variant van de ziekte van Huntington. *Ned. T. Geneesk.* **104**, 1625–1627.

Meggendorfer, F. (1923). Die psychischen Störungen bei der Huntingtonschen Chorea, klinische und genealogische Untersuchungen. (Zugleich Mitteilung 11 neuer Huntington-Familien). *Z. ges. Neurol. Psychiat.* **87**, 1–49.

Meierhofer, M. (1937). Atypische Psychosen in einer Chorea-Huntington-Familie. *Mschr. Psychiat. Neurol.* **97**, 13–52.

Menzies, W. F. (1893). Cases of hereditary chorea (Huntington's disease). *J. ment. Sci.* **39**, 50–62.

Merritt, A. D., P. M. Conneally, N. F. Rahman & A. L. Drew (1969). Juvenile Huntington's chorea. *Progress in Neuro-Genetics*, eds. A. Barbeau & J. R. Brunette, Vol. 1, pp. 645–650. Excerpta Medica Foundation, Amsterdam.

Muncey, E. B. (1964). Huntington's chorea. (Mimeographed edition of the original field notes on which the publication of Davenport & Muncey (1916) was based. A copy was kindly supplied by Dr. Sheldon C. Reed, Dight Institute of Human Genetics, University of Michigan.)

Myrianthopoulos, N. C. & P. T. Rowley (1960). Monozygotic twins concordant for Huntington's chorea. *Arch. Neurol. (Minneap.)* **10**, 506–511.

Neumayer, E. & A. Rett (1966). Ein Choreasippe mit rigider Form. *Wien. Z. Nervenheilk.* **23**, 74–83.

Oepen, H., H. J. Landzettel, R. Streletzki & I. von Koppenfels (1963). Statistische Befunde zur Klinik der Huntingtonsche Chorea. *Arch. Psychiat. Nervenkr.* **204**, 11–24.

Oliver, J. E. (1970). Huntington's chorea in Northamptonshire. *Brit. J. Psychiat.* **116**, 241–253.

Oltman, J. E. & S. Friedman (1961). Comments on Huntington's chorea. *Dis. nerv. Syst.* **22**, 313–319.

Ørbeck, A. L. & T. Quelprud (1954). *Setesdalsrykka (Chorea Progressiva Hereditaria).* J. Dybwad, Oslo.

Pache, H. D. (1953). *Mschr. Kinderheilk.* **101**, 504.

Panse, F. (1942). Der Erbchorea. *Sammlung Psychiatrischer und Neurologischer Einzeldarstellung*, Band 18. G. Thieme, Berlin.

Parker, N. (1958). Observations on Huntington's chorea based on a Queensland survey. *Med. J. Aust.* **1**, 351–359.

Patzig, B. (1935). Vererbung von Bewegungsstörungen. *Z. indukt. Abstamm.-u. Vererb.-L.* **30**, 476.

Peretti, J. (1885). Ueber hereditäre choreatische Bewegungsstörungen. *Berl. klin. Wschr.* **22**, 824–827.

Petit, H. (1969). La maladie de Huntington. *Rapports 67e Session, Congrès de Psychiatrie et de Neurologie de Langue Francaise, Brussels.* Masson, Paris.

Pleydell, M. J. (1954). Huntington's chorea in Northamptonshire. *Brit. med. J.* **2**, 1121–1128.

Prosenz, P. (1966). Diskussion zum Vortrag Neumayer und Rett. *Wien Z. Nervenheilk.* **23**, 83–84.

Reisch, O. (1929). Studien an einer Huntington-Sippe. Ein Beitrag zur Symptomatologie verschiedener Stadien der Chorea Huntington. *Arch. Psychiat. Nervenkr.* **86**, 327–359.

Riggenbach, M. & A. Werthemann (1933). Untersuchungen bei einer Sippe von Huntington'scher Chorea. *Schweiz. Arch. Neurol. Psychiat.* **31**, 306–332.

Riggs, C. E. (1901). Three cases of hereditary chorea. *J. nerv. ment. Dis.* **28**, 519–521.

Rosenthal, C. (1927). Zur Symptomatologie und Fruhdiagnostik der Huntington'schen Krankheit, zugleich ein Beitrag zur klinischen Erbforschung (Degenerationserscheinungen und Konstitutionsanomalien in einem Huntingtonstamm). *Z. ges. Neurol. Psychiat.* **111**, 254–269.

Saginario, M., V. Corrente, S. Passeri & V. Bagnasco (1967). La variante rigida della corea di Huntington nell'eta' infanto-giovenile. *Sist. nerv.* **5**, 288–298.

Schiottz-Christensen, E. (1969). Chorea Huntington and epilepsy in monozygotic twins. *Europ. Neurol.* **2**, 250–255.

Schlesinger, H. (1892). Ueber einige seltenere Formen der Chorea. I. Chorea chronica hereditaria. II. Chorea chronica congenita. *Z. klin. Med.* **20**, 127–135.

Schönfelder, T. (1966). Kindliche Chorea Huntington. *Z. Kinderheilk.* **95**, 131–142.

Sjögren, T. (1935). Vererbungsmedizinische Untersuchungen über Huntingtons Chorea in einer schwedischen Bauernpopulation. *Z. menschl. Vererb.-u. Konstit.-Lehre.* **19**, 131–165.

Spillane, J. & R. Phillips (1937). Huntington's chorea in South Wales. *Quart. J. Med.* **6**, 403–423.

Starr, A. (1967). A disorder of rapid eye movements in Huntington's Chorea. *Brain* **90**, 545–564.

Stevens, D. & M. Parsonage (1969). Mutation in Huntington's chorea. *J. Neurol. Neurosurg. Psychiat.* **32**, 140–143.

Stone, S. (1932). Chronic progressive chorea (Huntington's disease). *New Engl. J. Med.* **207**, 974–983.

Stone, T. T. & E. I. Falstein (1939). Genealogical studies in Huntington's chorea. *J. nerv. ment. Dis.* **89**, 795–809.

Sumner, D. (1962). Amyotrophy in a family with Huntington's chorea. *Wld. Neurol.* **3**, 769–777.

Tay, C. H. (1970). Huntington's chorea: report of a Chinese family in Singapore. *J. med. Genet.* **7**, 41–43.

Tsuang, M. (1969). Huntington's chorea in a Chinese family. *J. med. Genet.* **6**, 354–356.

Worster-Drought, C. & I. M. Allen (1929). Huntington's chorea. *Brit. med. J.* **2**, 1149–1152.

Zolliker, A. (1949). Die chorea Huntington in der Schweiz. *Schweiz. Arch. Neurol. Psychiat.* **64**, 448–457.

No. of sibships	Neurological signs before psychiatric symptoms		Neurological signs coincident with psychiatric symptoms		Neurological signs after psychiatric symptoms		Reference	
	Males	Females	Males	Females	Males	Females		
1	1						Althaus	(1880)
1						1	Arai et al.	(1968)
1					1		Baron	(1950)
1	1	1					Beaubrun	(1963)
2				1		1	Becker	(1938)
1		1					Bell	(1934)
4			3	1	3	1	Bittenbender & Quadfasel	(1962)
7	1	1	2	1	2	3	Briebrecher	(1938)
1	1						Brothers	(1964)
14	4	3	1	4	2	3	Brothers & Meadows	(1955)
1				1			Buck	(1934)
1					1		Byers & Dodge	(1967)
2	1		3				Campbell et al.	(1961)
2	1		1				Chhuttani	(1955)
1			1			1	Curran	(1930)
3	4		3	1			Curschmann	(1908)
3			2	3			Delmas-Marsalet et al.	(1968)
1			1	2			De Marco & Testa	(1969)
1					1		Dewhurst	(1970)
3	1	1			2		Dewhurst & Oliver	(1970)
2	2						D'Ormea	(1904)
2	1	3					Entres	(1921)
1		1					Evans	(1908)
4	1				3	1	Frank	(1937)
3				1	2	2	Frets	(1943)
1		1					Gaule	(1932)
1						1	Geratovitsch	(1927)
4	2	1		3		1	Gezelle Meerburg	(1923)
1	2						Goldstein	(1913)
1			1		1	1	Goodman et al.	(1966)
1				1			Gröpl	(1968)
2				1		1	Hamilton	(1908)
1					1		Hempel	(1938)
2	1	1					Hoffmann	(1888)
1	1						Huber	(1887)
1		1					Huet	(1889)
1					1		Jervis	(1963)
1			1				Kalkhof & Ranke	(1913)
1		1					Kloos	(1938)
2		2					Lannois	(1888)
1	1	1	1				Leese et al.	(1952)
1					1		Mackenzie-van der Noordaa	(1960)
3				2	1	1	Meggendorfer	(1923)
1				1			Menzies	(1892)
27	11	7	5	7	2	4	Muncey	(1964)
1			1				Myrianthopoulos & Rowley	(1960)
1		1					Neumeyer & Rett	(1966)
5			1	1	4	6	Oliver	(1970)
1						1	Oltman & Friedman	(1961)
11	4	8	1	1	1	2	Ørbeck & Quelprud	(1954)
1				1			Pache	(1953)
9	1			2	4	2	Panse	(1942)
1						1	Parker	(1958)

No. of sibships	Neurological signs before psychiatric symptoms		Neurological signs coincident with psychiatric symptoms		Neurological signs after psychiatric symptoms		Reference	
	Males	Females	Males	Females	Males	Females		
2	1	1		1			Peretti	(1885)
5			3	1	1	1	Petit	(1969)
6		4		1	1	3	Pleydell	(1954)
1				1	1		Prosenz	(1966)
2		1				2	Reisch	(1929)
1			1				Riggenbach & Werthemann	(1933)
1		1					Riggs	(1901)
1				1			Rosenthal	(1927)
1				2			Saginario et al.	(1967)
1				2			Schiottz-Christensen	(1969)
1						2	Schlesinger	(1892)
4	1	1	2	2			Schönfelder	(1966)
11	8	8	2	1	1		Sjögren	(1935)
4		1	2	1		3	Spillane & Phillips	(1937)
3			1				Starr	(1967)
1	2	1					Stevens & Parsonage	(1969)
1			1				Stone	(1932)
2		1	1				Stone & Falstein	(1939)
1			2			1	Sumner	(1962)
1	2						Tay	(1970)
1			3				Tsuang	(1969)
1		1					Worster-Drought & Allen	(1929)
2				1	1		Zolliker	(1949)
Total	58	56	45	49	41	43		

A genetic and statistical study of some sex-related factors in Huntington's disease

C. J. Brackenridge

The advantages that literature compilations possess over regional surveys are limited but they arise if the number of subjects *in toto* or in a subpopulation is too small for statistical analysis to be meaningful. For example, cases of Huntington's disease with onset in childhood occur so rarely that a very large population would need to be sampled if a study were to be based on an ascertainment from a single location.

Ever since Huntington (1872) recorded the impression that the disorder "is as common and is indeed, I believe, more common among men than women", sex-related factors in Huntington's disease have received the attention of many investigators. These have ranged from evidence of sex-limited genes modifying the onset age (Haldane 1936) to sex differences in psychopathological symptoms (Tamir, Whittier & Korenyi 1969).

The major anthology of published cases is that of Bell (1934) who assembled sibships published until 1932. Since then several studies incorporating extensive pedigree information have been completed, in

This work was supported by a grant from the National Health and Medical Research Council of Australia.

120

cluding those of Sjögren (1935), Panse (1942), Ørbeck & Quelprud (1954), and Pleydell (1954). In addition the field notes of Muncey (1964) have become available, so that a large body of data now exists for re-examining conclusions based on the material of Bell. The following genetic and statistical study of sex-dependent aspects of Huntington's disease is derived from the accessible world literature.

Material and Method

Sibships drawn without any known bias from published case reports and pedigrees were subjected to the following selection procedure. (A) Unless all members of a sibship were affected with Huntington's disease, only sibships succeeded by at least two generations were included. (B) If the clinical state of any members could not be definitely classified as affected or unaffected, the sibship was excluded. This applied to sibships containing members who died unaffected in childhood or early adulthood. (C) If the sex of the parent transmitting the disease was unknown, the sibship was excluded.

These precautions were intended to ensure inclusion of cases of late onset, to permit estimation of the segregation ratio, and to reduce the chances of misdiagnosis.

Of the 1,553 sibships originally assembled, 517 (33.3 %) conformed to the criteria and were therefore used as material for the study. The source, location, and time of publication of each are cited in Appendices I and II. The greatest single contribution were 144 sibships (27.9 % of the total) from Muncey (1964). Eighty sibships (15.5 % of the present material) were also contained in the monograph of Bell (1934). The number of generations intervening between the time of ascertainment and each sibship were distributed as follows.

No. of intervening generations	No. of sibships
0	84
1	105
2	198
3	101
4	28
7	1

Tests of independence and goodness of fit were made using the log likelihood ratio (G) test (Sokal & Rohlf 1969), the continuity correction of Yates being applied when necessary.

Results and Discussion

Sex Incidence

The composition of sibships containing at least one person with Huntington's disease is presented in Table 1. The mean sibship size was 3.12. The sex ratio was 1.09 for unaffected subjects and 1.13 for affected subjects; the latter value differed significantly from unity but not from the sex ratio for unaffected persons. Neither displayed significant heterogeneity when the sex ratio was determined for all sibship sizes. The male preponderance was higher among procreators, being 1.22 for 517 parents and 1.37 for 358 grandparents who transmitted the disorder to the sibships described here. Ratios found in community surveys range from 0.72 (Reed & Chandler 1958) to 1.19 (Entres 1921).

Segregation Ratios

In kindreds segregating for a dominant trait, complete ascertainment of a population for the trait is usually carried out through an affected parent. However, in sibships published in the literature the methods of ascertainment must be diverse. It was therefore interesting to estimate segregation ratios for several different hypothetical modes of

Table 1

Composition of affected sibships

Sibship size	No. of sibships with no. of affected									No. of sibships	No. of affected males	No. of affected females	No. of unaffected males	No. of unaffected females	Total no. of siblings
	1	2	3	4	5	6	7	8	9						
1	176									176	96	80	0	0	176
2	19	81								100	94	87	10	9	200
3	10	13	43							66	86	79	20	13	198
4	3	15	16	22						56	87	82	27	28	224
5	6	9	13	5	4					37	51	52	43	39	185
6	3	4	8	6	4	5				30	61	47	40	32	180
7	2	0	4	4	3	5	0			18	36	39	28	23	126
8	0	1	0	2	1	5	0	0		9	30	15	14	13	72
9	0	1	4	4	3	1	0	0	0	13	29	22	31	35	117
10	0	0	1	0	0	1	0	1	0	4	11	8	12	9	40
11	0	1	0	0	0	2	0	1	1	5	18	13	12	12	55
12	0	0	0	0	0	1	0	0	0	1	1	5	3	3	12
13	0	0	0	1	0	0	0	0	0	1	2	2	4	5	13
14	0	0	0	1	0	0	0	0	0	1	1	3	4	6	14
Totals	219	126	89	45	15	20	0	2	1	517	603	534	248	227	1612

Table 2

Estimates and standard errors of segregation ratios derived from
hypothetical methods of ascertainment

Method of ascertainment	Reference	Segregation ratio
Complete ascertainment	Case 1, Smith (1958)	0.650 ± 0.012
Probability of ascertainment proportional to number affected	Case 2, Smith (1958)	0.566 ± 0.015
Constant probability of ascertainment per individual	Case 3, Smith (1958)	0.633 ± 0.017
Case 1, except that sibships with one affected only are not considered	Haldane (1949)	0.622 ± 0.017
Case 2, except that sibships with one affected only are not considered	Haldane (1949)	0.559 ± 0.018

ascertainment to see which provided the closest fit to expectation. Table 2 lists the results calculated from some of the commoner models.

The greatest disparity was obtained on the assumption that ascertainment was complete. In this procedure, case 1 in the terminology of Smith (1958), it is postulated that sampling of sibships is at random and that the probability of inclusion is independent of their composition (except that at least one person is affected). The closest fit was obtained in a possibility considered by Haldane (1949). If there is reason to believe that single-membered sibships are less likely to be reported than those containing several affected persons, there is justification for estimating segregation ratios from sibships containing at least two affected cases. Inspection of Table 1 reveals that the distributions in sibships of sizes 2, 3, and 4 are biased by a high proportion of affected persons; grounds therefore exist for further supposing that the probability of selection varies directly with the number of affected siblings. The estimate of 0.559 derived from these assumptions comes closest to the theoretical value of 0.5, so that they are likely to be factors in the reporting of genetic information.

Estimates of the segregation ratio from community studies are also subject to difficulties due to diagnostic uncertainty, late onset of symptoms, and early death. In spite of these, Sjögren (1935) in northern Sweden, Panse (1942) in the Rhineland, and Reed & Chandler (1958) in Michigan obtained satisfactory agreement with the expected value in each of their analyses based on complete ascertainment.

Test for Familial Sex-Limitation

To determine whether the proportion of affected sib-pairs of like sex differed appreciably from the proportion of affected sib-pairs of unlike sex, frequencies of the three possible pairings between affected males and females were counted. Of 1,201 pairs, 631 were of like sex and 570 were of unlike sex (Table 3). Although the difference is not significant ($G = 3.07$, $P > 0.05$), it was sufficiently suggestive to warrant testing for familial sex-limitation. When the data were extended to involve all sibship members, analysis of Table 3 by the procedure of Penrose & Watson (1945) showed that the weighted L-value (an index of limitation) of 5.21 did not exceed twice the standard sampling error of ± 3.44. Thus there is no appreciable tendency for sibships affected with the disease to have an excess of like-sexed members.

Table 3

Numbers of sib-pairs of affected and unaffected persons

Type of sib	Affected males	Affected females	Unaffected males	Unaffected females
Affected males	376			
Affected females	570	255		
Unaffected males	351	368	169	
Unaffected females	348	321	325	159

Table 4

Distribution of offspring among affected parental-grandparental lines

Type of offspring	Father-grandfather	Father-grandmother	Mother-grandfather	Mother-grandmother	Test of goodness of fit to equal proportions	
					G	P
Affected sons	130	77	86	74	20.66	< 0.001
Affected daughters	106	79	108	72	11.28	< 0.02
Affected offspring	236	156	194	146	26.95	< 0.001
Unaffected sons	60	30	24	28	20.80	< 0.001
Unaffected daughters	35	32	32	40	1.21	> 0.7
Unaffected offspring	95	62	56	68	12.04	< 0.01
Total offspring	331	218	250	214	33.37	< 0.001

Test for Partial Sex-Linkage

The data in Table 4 reveal that the father-grandfather line dominates the possible lines of transmission, the divergence from proportions of 1:1:1:1 being significant for all types of offspring except unaffected daughters. A preliminary test of partial sex-linkage was performed according to Haldane (1936). In this method the number of affected persons of the same sex as the affected grandparent is added to the number of unaffected persons of unlike sex to the unaffected grandparent and the total is expressed as a proportion of the total offspring of affected fathers. The value of 0.499 obtained is very close to the expected value of 0.5 for absence of linkage.

In a previous analysis carried out on the material of Bell (1934), evidence supporting linkage was derived by Haldane (1936). The minimum age at which offspring of affected persons were reckoned as normal was taken to be 30 years in his results in Table 5, which lists the frequencies of Oepen (1965) and the present study for comparison. However a number of considerations led Haldane to reject the hypothesis in favour of sex-limited modifying genes. He argued that if there are modifiers in a family increasing the onset age in females, there will be an excess of males among the affected and of females among the normal. This would account for the numbers he obtained. (Parenthetically, this is an unlikely explanation since no published work has yet demonstrated a significantly higher onset age for females.)

Under the present conditions of selection, all siblings except some who had already died from Huntington's disease were of grandparental age and the number falsely classified as normal due to late onset should be relatively low. Consequently the effect observed by Haldane should not be found.

124

Type of offspring	Fathers-sons	Fathers-daughters	Mothers-sons	Mothers-daughters	Reference
Affected	344	286	259	248	Present study
Unaffected	143	119	105	108	
Affected	128	91	79	106	Haldane (1941)
Unaffected	77	118	61	56	
Affected	425	414	306	404	Oepen (1965)
Unaffected	563	514	469	445	

The present findings in Table 5 show that this is so; males preponderate among affected and unaffected siblings. The divergence from equal proportions was significant for parent-affected offspring pairs (G = 18.93, P < 0.001) but not for pairs of parents and unaffected offspring (G = 7.31, P > 0.05). An important feature of the three sets of results in Table 5 is the excess of father-son pairs among affected persons. Among the unaffected, mother-daughter pairs are least frequent or next to least frequent. The excess of sons over daughters of affected fathers observed in the present investigation agrees with the results of Oepen. In contrast the sex ratios among maternal offspring are appreciably different; both Haldane and Oepen found more affected daughters than affected sons and more unaffected sons than unaffected daughters, but this was not evident in the literature survey.

Some possible reasons for the predominance of fathers and sons were next considered and examined as follows.

(1) Affected fathers produce sibships with an excess of males. This simple hypothesis is excluded by the finding that the mean number of sons of 284 affected fathers (1.72) is not significantly higher (G = 0.60, P > 0.5) than the mean number of sons of 233 affected mothers (1.56). When sons were subdivided into healthy and affected, the lack of significance persisted.

(2) Affected females have a lower fitness than affected males. If this gave rise to a relatively high female perinatal mortality, it could provide a plausible explanation of the data. Unfortunately too few details of stillbirths were found to test the hypothesis, so that evidence on this point can only be derived from a field survey. If postnatal death resulted from reduced fitness, this would not explain the findings because of the selection procedure operating against inclusion of cases of death in infancy. However, under conditions of ascertainment different from those applying here, differential mortality is a definite possibility. In their Michigan survey, Reed & Neel (1959) reported that the proportion of deaths among children of affected males was significantly lower than among those of affected females and pointed out that, if the difference is real, it is not surprising since the mother is probably more important to the survival of an infant than is the father.

(3) Sons of affected males have a greater fertility than other types of subjects. This possibility is difficult to test because unmarried and childless persons were not always distinguished in the literature from those for whom no information was available. However, for those known to have reproduced, an analysis of variance provided no evidence of heterogeneity among the four types of descent (F = 0.17 for 3 and 615 d.f.). It would therefore require a disproportionate number of unmarried or childless cases between the sexes to account

for the ascendancy of the male line on the basis of fertility.

Two other investigations bearing on this point reached different conclusions. With respect to affected subjects, single or married, Reed & Neel (1959) found that 47 of 120 males (39.2 %) produced no live-births whereas 30 of 137 females (21.9 %) produced no live-births. The difference is significant (P < 0.005). On the other hand, Wendt, Solth & Landzettel (1961) found that 293 of 1,157 males (25.3 %) and 336 of 1,233 females (27.3 %) were childless. This difference is not significant. As the data of Oepen (1965) were based on the material of Wendt et al. (1961), sex-dependent differences in fertility could not have been responsible for the high frequency of patrilineal transmission he reported.

(4) An artefact due to sampling bias is responsible. This is unlikely insofar as the material of Oepen was free from known selection bias and had a sex ratio of 0.89, properties in contrast to those of the present study, yet the excess of affected pairs of fathers and sons occurs also in his results.

No evidence of heterogeneity was obtained when the frequencies of the literature survey in Table 5 were analysed according to sibship size and the number of generations between the time of ascertainment and the sibship of interest.

(5) Quantitative factors such as differences in onset age create conditions favouring the male line of descent. These possibilities are explored in the following sections.

Age at Onset of Symptoms

Among the factors which could produce an excess of single or childless females and thereby promote patrilineal descent is an earlier onset age of women. A lower age at death might also serve as an index, particularly in subjects whose age at onset was unknown or could not be estimated accurately because of insidious development of symptoms.

The early signs of Huntington's disease may be characterized by abnormal behaviour or motor impairment. Some investigators have related onset age to the appearance of choreic movements (Reed & Chandler 1958) while others have dated it from any symptoms attributable to the disorder (Bell 1934, Panse 1942, Wendt et al. 1959, Dewhurst, Oliver & McKnight 1970). In Table 6 none of the differences between males and females is significant. In the present material the onset age of all subjects (33.84 ± 0.71 years) and for females is the lowest of any tabulated. Reed & Chandler (1958) and Dewhurst et al. (1970) were the only authors to report a higher onset age in females than in males.

Table 6

Mean age at onset of symptoms in different surveys

Source	Males		Females		Total	
	Number	Mean	Number	Mean	Number	Mean
Bell (1934)	256	36.1	197	35.2	460	35.5
Panse (1942)	225	36.5	221	35.7	446	36.2
Ørbeck & Quelprud (1954)	48	42.3	61	37.8	109	39.8
Reed & Chandler (1958)	86	34.6	118	35.9	204	35.3
Wendt et al. (1959)	377	44.3	385	43.7	762	44.0
Petit (1969)	56	41.1	69	39.3	125	40.0
Dewhurst et al. (1970)	55	37.8	47	39.9	102	38.8
Present study	183	34.8	161	32.8	344	33.8

To avoid the error incurred by considering subjects born too soon before the time of ascertainment and thereby acquiring a disproportionately large number of cases of early onset, Wendt et al. (1959) made their estimate on cases born during the period 1870 to 1899. The effect of this precaution is, like the present study, to ensure that persons were essentially of grandparental age and unlikely to develop the disease later. It is therefore surprising that the ages determined by Wendt et al. are significantly higher than those found here. A possible reason for the discrepancy is that the sample of Wendt et al. may have comprised a smaller proportion of cases of the 'juvenile' and 'Westphal' variants which have a lower onset age than 'classical' cases. (According to Bittenbender & Quadfasel (1962) the mean onset age in the Westphal type is about 22 years.) This hypothesis is supported by a comparison of percentages of juvenile cases with onset of symptoms at 20 years or less. Seventeen of the 762 subjects (2.2 %) of Wendt et al. and 59 of the present 340 subjects (17.4 %) were in this category. The difference is highly significant ($G = 74.22$, $P < 0.001$). Bruyn (1968) has estimated the proportion of juvenile cases to be 5 to 10 % of all subjects with Huntington's disease; the excess of present cases is probably an over-representation due to their exceptional interest.

The high incidence of juvenile subjects could also account for the ascendancy of the male line. Bruyn (1968) concluded from a survey of 150 published cases that there is a preponderance of females to males of between 1.5:1 and 2:1 and that in about 70 % of the instances the patients received the gene from the father. The 59 present cases were drawn from 48 sibships of whom the transmitting parent was the father 33 times and the mother 15 times. The difference between this proportion and the

sex ratio (251/218) of the affected parents of the remaining sibships having no juvenile cases is of borderline significance. However, when juvenile subjects and their progenitors were excluded from the results in Tables 4 and 5, no significant difference was introduced and the order of frequency of the parental-grandparental lines and parent-sib pairs was not disturbed.

The possibility remained that an appreciable proportion of cases of relatively early onset (including all juvenile, most Westphal, and some classical cases), which would be more noteworthy for purposes of publication than those of later onset, arise from paternal transmission of the abnormal gene. This could then explain the male preponderance. The mean onset ages of persons with affected fathers and mothers were therefore calculated and are compared in Table 7. No significant differences emerged from an analysis of variance and there was no evidence of interaction between sex of parents and sex of offspring.

Oepen (1965) found a tendency in the first half of life for more children of affected fathers to show symptoms and die than children of affected mothers. This trend is apparent in Table 7, being more marked for daughters than for sons, but the resulting heterogeneity is not significant.

The suggestion that affected fathers induce a shift to a younger age at onset in their offspring was apparently first made by Merritt, Conneally, Rahman & Drew (1969). It was tested by Jones & Phillips (1970) who searched the records of all state mental hospitals in Pennsylvania and found the mean onset age of 46 paternal cases to be 37.5 years and of 84 maternal cases to be 40.2 years. In agreement with the present result, the difference was not significant.

The trend towards an earlier onset age for daughters is unlikely to be a factor in the predominance of the male line since

Table 7

Relation of mean onset age of affected offspring to sex of transmitting parent

Offspring	Fathers		Mothers	
	Number	Mean	Number	Mean
Sons	155	34.61 ± 1.30	68	35.07 ± 1.63
Daughters	95	31.08 ± 1.30	66	35.21 ± 1.49
Total	210	33.01 ± 0.93	134	35.14 ± 1.10

Table 8

Mean age at death in different surveys

Source	Males		Females		Total	
	Number	Mean	Number	Mean	Number	Mean
Bell (1934)	191	53.6	158	52.6	349	53.1
Panse (1942)	247	52.2	226	52.2	473	52.2
Ørbeck & Quelprud (1954)	52	56.2	65	55.0	117	55.5
Reed & Chandler (1958)	125	53.1	137	54.1	262	53.6
Wendt et al. (1961)	783	54.2	791	53.6	1574	54.0
Brothers (1964)	66	51.2	57	51.7	123	51.4
Husquinet (1969)	105	53.7	126	54.5	231	54.1
Petit (1969)	71	55.3	70	56.0	141	55.6
Dewhurst et al. (1970)	55	51.7	47	55.5	102	53.5
Present study	218	52.9	185	50.2	403	51.7

affected males also descend largely from affected fathers and grandfathers (Tables 4 and 5) and, of females known to have reproduced, the mean number of offspring of 164 paternal cases (4.24 ± 0.23) was not significantly different from that of 142 maternal cases (4.12 ± 0.23).

Age at Death

Age at death can be fixed with higher precision than age at onset but suffers from the uncertainty that it may not be directly attributable to the pathology of Huntington's disease. The average age at death (51.65 ± 0.81 years for 403 persons) was not affected by the sex of the subject in agreement with results of previous surveys (Table 8). The mean value found for females was lower than those reported elsewhere. Parental descent exercised no significant influence (Table 9).

Duration of Symptoms

The distributions of the ages at onset and death were essentially normal but length of illness was distributed with a positive skew. Conversion of the data to logarithms yielded a more Gaussian distribution. After transformation, duration of symptoms was independent of the sex of the patient in agreement with previous investigations (Table 10), but the present means were lower in magnitude. This is because the logarithmic conversion reduced the mean values by about 2.5 years from what they would be if a normal distribution were assumed. The mean value for 191 subjects was 11.92 years, the 95 % confidence limits being 10.86 and 13.08 years.

When the sex of the transmitting parent was considered, paternal cases had a significantly shorter span of illness than maternal cases (F = 7.52 for 1 and 187 d.f., P < 0.01). This was due chiefly to the contribu-

128

Table 9

Relation of mean age at death of affected offspring to sex of transmitting parent

Offspring	Fathers		Mothers	
	Number	Mean	Number	Mean
Sons	126	52.52 ± 1.51	92	53.36 ± 1.59
Daughters	100	49.28 ± 1.63	85	51.36 ± 1.75
Total	226	51.08 ± 1.11	177	52.40 ± 1.18

Table 10

Mean duration of symptoms in years in different surveys

Source	Males		Females		Total	
	Number	Mean	Number	Mean	Number	Mean
Panse (1942)	143	13.9	128	13.1	271	13.4
Reed & Chandler (1958)	65	15.8	88	15.9	153	15.9
Wendt et al. (1960)	109	12.2	119	13.5	228	12.9
Petit (1969)	28	14.1	37	14.6	65	14.4
Dewhurst et al. (1970)	55	13.9	47	15.6	102	14.7
Present study	105	12.2	86	11.6	191	11.9

Table 11

Relation of mean duration of symptoms (in years) of affected offspring to sex of
transmitting parent

(Values in parentheses are 95 % confidence limits of the lognormal distributions)

Offspring	Fathers*		Mothers*	
	Number	Mean	Number	Mean
Sons	63	10.61 (8.98–12.53)	42	14.90 (12.31–18.03)
Daughters	47	10.80 (8.88–13.14)	39	12.74 (10.40–15.60)
Total	110	10.69 (9.44–12.12)	81	13.81 (12.04–15.84)

* Differences among subjects attributable to sex of parents adjusted for sex of offspring are significant at the
1 % level

tion made by sons (Table 11). There was no detectable interaction between the sex of subjects and the sex of their parents. The role of the sex of an affected parent in relation to length of illness of offspring bears upon the heritability of this quantity and suggests that sex is a relevant variable in parent-offspring correlations.

Influence of Time of Ascertainment
If age at death is ascertained for a late generation of a kindred affected with Huntington's disease, a bias could be created in favour of those who die relatively young. Conversely, the mean age at death of an earlier generation could be biased by relatively late deaths because of the reduced fitness for parenthood of subjects with early onset of symptoms. Therefore if parents are ascertained through their children, ages at onset and at death are likely to increase from present to past generations. This prob-

lem has been discussed by Wendt *et al.* (1959, 1961) in relation to their West German survey.

Analyses of variance were carried out on ages at onset and death and duration of illness of affected persons up to four generations preceding the time of ascertainment. The results in Table 12 confirm the expected trend. The increase in age at death with increasing number of intervening generations slightly outstrips the increase in age at onset so that the duration of symptoms of recent cases is shorter than that of their antecedents. The heterogeneity is significant for age at onset ($F = 30.97$ for 4 and 339 d.f., $P < 0.001$) and age at death ($F = 24.17$ for 4 and 397 d.f., $P < 0.001$) but not for length of illness ($F = 1.13$ for 4 and 186 d.f., $P > 0.2$). It is clear that under conditions other than complete ascertainment, such as ascertainment of parents through children, ages at onset and death will appear to vary from generation to generation and the phenomenon of anticipation is produced. Attention has been drawn by earlier investigators to this artefact (Davenport & Muncey 1916, Bell 1942).

When affected subjects were distributed among generations according to their sex and to the sex of their transmitting parent, there was no evidence of heterogeneity from G-tests of independence. The dif-

ference found in duration of illness in Table 11 was therefore not due to the effect described here.

Influence of Sibship Size

The possible effect of sibship size on aspects of the disease was examined and the results are summarized in Table 13. It can be seen that the mean onset ages of members of small sibships is appreciably lower than for those in sibships containing four or more persons. The heterogeneity is significant ($F = 7.35$ for 7 and 336 d.f., $P < 0.001$) for mean age at onset but not for age at death ($F = 0.47$ for 7 and 395 d.f., $P > 0.2$) or for duration of symptoms ($F = 0.94$ for 7 and 183 d.f., $P > 0.2$). Distribution of affected persons in relation to sex and sex of affected parent was independent of sibship size; heterogeneity was therefore not a contributing factor to the difference reported in Table 11.

The decision by parents to limit the number of their offspring after the birth of an unfit child is relevant only to the few cases of very early onset of symptoms. Similarly the hypothesis that onset age is proportionate to the number of other affected members of a sibship is unattractive. It seems more likely that the onset age of a parent will be related to the number of offspring produced; many small sibships will be due

Table 12

Relation of age at onset, age at death, and duration of symptoms to the number of generations from the time of ascertainment

Number of intervening generations	Age at onset		Age at death		Duration of symptoms	
	Number of persons	Mean age (years)	Number of persons	Mean age (years)	Number of persons	Time* (years)
0	69	21.54 ± 1.57	41	37.63 ± 2.88	31	10.57 (8.38–13.35)
1	73	31.93 ± 1.19	56	41.39 ± 1.28	25	11.62 (9.16–14.76)
2	143	37.80 ± 0.93	175	53.02 ± 1.07	89	11.71 (10.02–13.50)
3	48	41.21 ± 1.65	96	57.84 ± 1.67	36	12.41 (10.30–14.94)
4	11	40.09 ± 3.07	34	60.65 ± 2.37	10	17.25 (10.64–27.99)

* Values in parentheses are 95 % confidence limits of the lognormal distributions.

Table 13

Relation of age at onset, age at death, and duration of symptoms to sibship size

Sibship size	Age at onset		Age at death		Duration of symptoms	
	Number of persons	Mean age (years)	Number of persons	Mean age (years)	Number of persons	Time* (years)
1	65	27.52 ± 1.77	66	51.03 ± 2.15	28	12.05 (9.49–15.31)
2	69	29.88 ± 1.68	60	49.53 ± 2.35	28	11.65 (9.29–14.61)
3	52	31.92 ± 1.74	54	51.17 ± 2.58	23	12.19 (9.09–16.36)
4	48	38.23 ± 1.28	75	53.51 ± 1.74	35	13.66 (11.44–16.30)
5	30	40.30 ± 2.62	44	53.68 ± 2.62	21	9.43 (6.30–14.11)
6	34	39.38 ± 1.67	44	51.20 ± 2.10	27	11.13 (8.86–13.98)
7–8	18	39.33 ± 2.80	30	50.13 ± 2.44	11	10.11 (5.45–18.75)
9–14	28	37.14 ± 1.76	30	52.83 ± 1.98	18	14.20 (10.38–19.40)

* Values in parentheses are 95 % confidence limits of the lognormal distributions.

to decreased parental fitness resulting from onset of symptoms in early adulthood. If a significant correlation exists between parent and offspring for age at onset, then the members of small sibships would display symptoms earlier than those of large sibships. Some support for this suggestion can be drawn from previous work. Wendt *et al.* (1961) found a correlation coefficient of 0.181 between onset age and number of children of 1,394 affected persons. This is significant, as is also the correlation coefficient of 0.593 between onset ages of 153 pairs of parents and offspring (P < 0.001) reported by Bell (1942).

The hypothesis was tested directly from the present material by comparing ages at onset of parents producing small sibships of sizes 1 to 3 with those producing large sibships of sizes 4 to 14. The mean age at onset of 29 parents of large sibships (43.45 ± 1.84 years) was significantly later (P < 0.02) than the age at onset of 67 parents of small sibships (36.75 ± 1.48 years). This was due principally to the later onset age (P < 0.02) of 18 mothers of large sibships (42.56 ± 2.31 years) compared with that of 30 mothers of small sibships (33.90 ± 2.31 years). The hypothesis is therefore supported by these results.

Conclusions

None of the variables for which data were available has led to a satisfactory explanation of the high frequency of patrilineal transmission of Huntington's disease. The tacit assumption throughout this work that the disorder is a homogeneous entity may be an oversimplification which masks the factors responsible. In the following contribution (Brackenridge 1971) the effects of separating out some clinical variables are examined.

References

Althaus, J. (1880). Chorea mit Epilepsie gepaart. *Arch. Psychiat. Nervenkr.* **10**, 139.

Arai, Y., A. Goto, T. Majima, K. Murofushi & H. Narabayashi (1968). Two cases of Huntington's chorea. Clinical and neuropathological studies of a typical and an atypical form in a family. *Clin. Neurol. (Tokyo)* **8**, 635.

Ballentine, E. P. (1912). Review of six cases of hereditary chorea. *N.Y. St. J. Med.* **12**, 644.

Barbeau, A., C. Coiteux, J. G. Trudeau & G. Fullum (1964). La chorée de Huntington chez les Canadiens Francais. Étude preliminaire. *Un méd. Can.* **93**, 1178.

Baron, G. (1950). Contribution à l'étude clinique et génétique des chorées chroniques progressives familiales maladie de Huntington et états Huntingtonniers. Thesis, Faculté de Médecine de Paris.

Beaubrun, M. H. (1963). Huntington's chorea in Trinidad. *W. Indian med. J.* **12**, 39.

Becker, G. (1938). Beitrag zur Klinik und Genealogie der Huntingtonschen Chorea. *Allg. Z. Psychiat.* **107**, 193.

Bell, J. (1934). Nervous disease and muscular dystrophies. Part I. Huntington's chorea. *The Treasury of Human Inheritance,* ed. R. A. Fisher & L. S. Penrose. Cambridge University Press, London.

Bell, J. (1942). On the age of onset and age at death in hereditary muscular dystrophy with some observations bearing on the question of antedating. *Ann. Eugen.* **11**, 272.

Bellamy, W. E. & Green, N. (1961). Huntington's chorea. *N. C. med. J.* **22**, 409.

Bickford, J. A. R. & R. M. Ellison (1953). The high incidence of Huntington's chorea in the duchy of Cornwall. *J. ment. Sci.* **99**, 291.

Bittenbender, J. B. & F. A. Quadfasel (1962). Rigid and akinetic forms of Huntington's chorea. *Arch. Neurol. (Chic.)* **7**, 275.

Böhm, J. (1938). Die Chorea-Huntington-Sippe Fellhauer. Dissertation, University of Heidelberg.

Bower, J. L. (1890). Notes on some cases of chorea tremor. *J. nerv. ment. Dis.* **15**, 131.

Brackenridge, C. J. (1971). The relation of type of initial symptoms and line of transmission to ages at onset and death in Huntington's disease. *Clin. Genet.* **2**, 287.

Briebrecher, G. (1938). Chorea Huntington-Sippe. Dissertation, University of Bonn.

Brothers, C. R. D. (1949). The history and incidence of Huntington's chorea in Tasmania. *Proc. roy. Aust. Coll. Phycns.* **4**, 48.

Brothers, C. R. D. (1964). Huntington's chorea in Victoria and Tasmania. *J. neurol. Sci.* **1**, 405.

Brothers, C. R. D. & A. W. Meadows (1955). An investigation of Huntington's chorea in Victoria. *J. ment. Sci.* **101**, 548.

Bruyn, G. W. (1968). Huntington's chorea. Historical, clinical and laboratory synopsis. *Handbook of Clinical Neurology,* ed. P. J. Vinken & G. W. Bruyn, Vol. 6, p. 298. North-Holland Publishing Co., Amsterdam.

Buck, C. A. (1934). Huntington's chorea, with the report of a case. *Canad. med. Ass. J.* **31**, 178.

Byers, R. K. & J. A. Dodge (1967). Huntington's chorea in children. Report of four cases. *Neurology (Minneap.)* **17**, 587.

Calkins, R. A. & M. W. van Allen (1967). Huntington's chorea *J. Iowa St. med. Soc.* **57**, 336.

Campbell, A. M. G., B. Corner, R. M. Norman & H. Urich (1961). The rigid form of Huntington's disease. *J. Neurol. Neurosurg. Psychiat.* **24**, 71.

Chamberlain, L. C. (1943). Abstract of clinical history of case 2. *New Orleans med. surg. J.* **96**, 57.

Chandler, J. H., T. E. Reed & R. N. De Jong (1960). Huntington's chorea in Michigan. III. Clinical observations. *Neurology (Minneap.)* **10**, 148.

Clarke, C. K. & J. W. MacArthur (1924). Four generations of hereditary chorea. *J. Hered.* **15**, 303.

Cronin, E. J. (1943). Huntington's chorea. *N. Z. med. J.* **42**, 231.

Curran, D. (1930). Huntington's chorea without choreiform movements. *J. Neurol. Psychopath.* **10**, 305.

Curschmann, H. (1908). Eine neue Chorea-Huntingtonfamilie. *Dtsch. Z. Nervenheilk.* **35**, 293.

Dana, C. L. (1895). The pathology of hereditary chorea. Report of a case with autopsy; record of anomalies in a degenerate brain. *J. nerv. ment. Dis.* **20**, 565.

Davenport, C. B. & E. B. Muncey (1916). Huntington's chorea in relation to heredity and eugenics. *Amer. J. Insan.* **73**, 195.

Delmas-Marsalet, P., M. Bourgeois, C. Vital & X. Fontanges (1968). Formes rigides de la maladie de Huntington (étude d'une famille avec un cas anatomo-clinique). *Rev. neurol.* **118**, 273.

Dercum, F. X. (1892). Adult chorea. *Int. Clin.* **3**, 292.

Dewhurst, K. & J. Oliver (1970). Huntington's disease of young people. *Europ. Neurol.* **3**, 278.

Dewhurst, K., J. E. Oliver & A. L. McKnight (1970). Socio-psychiatric consequences of Huntington's disease. *Brit. J. Psychiat.* **116**, 255.

D'Ormea, A. (1904). Una famiglia coreica. *Rif. med.* **20**, 313.

Dow, D. S. (1960). Huntington's chorea. Differentiated from Wilson's disease with report of unusual case. *Rocky Mtn. med. J.* **57**, 44.

El-Garem, O. (1958). The first record of three families of Huntington's chorea in Egypt. *Alexandria med. J.* **4**, 364.

Entres, J. L. (1921). Zur Klinik und Vererbung der Huntington'schen Chorea. *Monogr. ges. geb. Neurol. Psychiat.* Heft 37. Springer-Verlag, Berlin.

Entres, J. L. (1940). Der Erbveitstanz. *Handbuch der Erbkrankheiten,* ed. A. Gütt, Band 3, p. 243.

Evans, J. J. W. (1908). Observations on a case of Huntington's chorea. *Lancet* **2**, 940.

Ewald, C. A. (1884). Zwei Falle choreatischer Zwangsbewegungen mit ausgesprochener Hereditat. *Z. klin. Med.* **7**, 51.

Facklam, F. C. (1898). Beitrage zur Lehre vom Wesen der Huntington'schen Chorea. *Arch. Psychiat. Nervenkr.* **30**, 137.

Finn, R. (1970). The three-century history of an Iowa family with Huntington's chorea. *J. Iowa St. med. Soc.* **60**, 89.

Frank, W. (1937). Untersuchungen über Chorea Huntington an Hand von 19 Fällen unter besonderer Berucksichtigung der Erblichkeit und der Fruhsymptome. *Psychiat. neurol. Wschr.* **39**, 51.

Fraser, L. A. & Updike, M. E. (1969). Huntington's chorea: a case investigation. *J. med. Soc. N. J.* **66**, 256.

Frets, G. P. (1943). De erfelijkheid bij 15 lijders aan chronische, progressieve chorea (Huntington), die in de jaren 1914–1941 in de psychiatrische inrichting "Maasoord" verpleegd zijn. *Genetica* **23**, 465.

Freund, C. S. (1925). Zur vererbung der Huntington'schen Chorea. *Z. ges. Neurol. Psychiat.* **99**, 333.

Gale, F. & J. H. Bennett (1969). Huntington's chorea in a South Australian community of Aboriginal descent. *Med. J. Aust.* **2**, 482.

Gaule, A. (1932). Das Auftreten der Chorea Huntington in einer Familie der Nordostschweiz. *Schweiz. Arch. Neurol. Psychiat.* **29**, 90.

Geratovitsch, M. (1927). Über Erblichkeitsuntersuchungen bei der Huntington'schen Krankheit. *Arch. Psychiat. Nervenkr.* **80**, 513.

Gezelle Meerburg, G. F. (1923). Bijdrage, naar aanleiding van een anatomisch en genealogisch onderzoek tot de kennis van de chorea Huntingtonea. *Thesis,* University of Utrecht.

Goldstein, M. (1913). Ein kasuistischer Beitrag zur Chorea chronica hereditaria. *Münch. med. Wschr.* **60**, 1659.

Greppin, L. (1892). Ueber einen Fall Huntington'scher Chorea. *Arch. Psychiat. Nervenkr.* **24**, 155.

Gröpl, H. (1968). Chorea Huntington im Kindesalter. *Z. Kinderheilk.* **103**, 45.

Haldane, J. B. S. (1936). A search for incomplete sex-linkage in man. *Ann. Eugen.* **7**, 28.

Haldane, J. B. S. (1941). The relative importance of principal and modifying genes in determining some human diseases. *J. Genet.* **41**, 149.

Haldane, J. B. S. (1949). A test for homogeneity of records of familial abnormalities. *Ann. Eugen.* **14**, 339.

Hamilton, A. S. (1908). A report of twenty-seven cases of chronic progressive chorea. *Amer. J. Insan.* **64**, 403.

Hansotia, P., C. S. Cleeland & R. W. M. Chun (1968). Juvenile Huntington's chorea. *Neurology (Minneap.)* **18**, 217.

Hanssen, O. (1914). Den Saetesdalske chorea St. Viti. *Med. Rev. (Bergen)* **31**, 569.

Harbinson, A. (1880). Sclerosis of the nervous centres, mainly cerebral. *Med. Press* **1**, 123.

Hattie, W. H. (1909). Huntington's chorea. *Amer. J. Insan.* **66**, 123.

Heathfield, K. W. G. (1967). Huntington's chorea. Investigation into the prevalence of this disease in the area covered by the North East Metropolitan Regional Hospital Board. *Brain* **90**, 203.

Hempel, H. C. (1938). Ein beitrag zur Huntingtonschen Erkrankung. *Z. ges. Neurol. Psychiat.* **160**, 563.

Hindringer, P. (1936). Eine neue Chorea Huntington-Sippe mit einer kurzen Zusammenstellung des gesamten Schrifttums der letzten 15 Jahre über Chorea Huntington. *Thesis,* University of Erlangen.

Hoffmann, J. (1888). Ueber Chorea chronica progressiva (Huntington'sche Chorea, Chorea hereditaria). *Virchows Arch. path. Anat.* **111**, 513.

Hogg, C. A. (1902). Two cases of Huntington's chorea, with a family history. *Aust. med. Gaz.* **21**, 400.

Huber, A. (1887). Chorea hereditaria der Erwachsenen (Huntington'sche Chorea). *Virchows Arch. path. Anat.* **108**, 267.

Huet, E. (1889). De la chorée chronique. *Thesis,* University of Paris.

Huntington, G. (1872). On chorea. *Med. surg. Reporter* **26**, 317.

Husquinet, H. (1969). La chorée de Huntington dans quatre provinces Belges. *Rapports 67e Session, Congrès de Psychiatrie et de Neurologie de Langue Francaise, Brussels.* Masson et Cie, Paris.

Jelliffe, S. E. & W. A. White (1917). *Diseases of the Nervous System,* 2nd ed. p. 29. Lea & Febiger, Philadelphia.

Jones, M. B. & C. R. Phillips (1970). Affected parent and age of onset in Huntington's chorea. *J. med. Genet.* **7**, 20.

Kloos, G. (1938). Gehaufte erbliche Taubheit in einer Huntington-Familie. *Münch. med. Wschr.* **85**, 94.

Laane, C. L. (1951). Den tidlige diagnose av chorea Huntington. *Nord. Med.* **45**, 835.

Lannois, M. (1888). Chorée hereditaire. *Rev. Med.* **8**, 645.

Lion, E. G. & E. Kahn (1938). Experiential aspects of Huntington's chorea. *Amer. J. Psychiat.* **95**, 717.

Lyon, I. W. (1863). Chronic hereditary chorea. *Amer. med. Times* **7**, 289.

Lyon, R. L. (1962). Huntington's chorea in the Moray Firth area. *Brit. med. J.* **1**, 1301.

Mackay, M. (1904). Hereditary chorea in eighteen members of a family, with a report of three cases. *Med. News N.Y.* **85**, 496.

Mackenzie-van der Noordaa, M.C. (1960). De door Westphal beschreven variant van de ziekte van Huntington. *Ned. Tijdschr. Geneesk.* **104**, 1625.

Meggendorfer, F. (1923). Die psychischen Störungen bei der Huntingtonschen Chorea, klinische und genealogische Untersuchungen. (Zugleich Mitteilung 11 neuer Huntington-familien.) *Z. ges. Neurol. Psychiat.* **87**, 1.

Menzies, W. F. (1892). Cases of hereditary chorea (Huntington's disease). *J. ment. Sci.* **38**, 560.

Menzies, W. F. (1893). Cases of hereditary chorea (Huntington's disease). *J. ment. Sci.* **39**, 50.

Merritt, A. D., P. M. Conneally, N. F. Rahman & A. L. Drew (1969). Juvenile Huntington's chorea. *Progress in Neuro-Genetics,* Vol. 1, p. 645. (Proc. 2nd Int. Congr. Neuro-Genetics and Neuro-Ophthalmology, Montreal, Sept. 1967.)

Mill, G. S. (1906). Huntington's chorea and heredity. *Brit. med. J.* **2**, 1215.

Minski, L. & E. Guttmann (1938). Huntington's chorea: a study of thirty four families. *J. ment. Sci.* **84**, 21.

Moody, P. A. (1967). *Genetics of Man,* p. 73. W. W. Norton & Co., New York.

Müller-Küppers, M. & K. Stenzel (1963). Zum Problem der Fruhmanifestation der Erbchorea. *Acta paedopsychiat.* **30**, 348.

Muncey, E. B. (1964). Huntington's chorea. (Mimeographed edition of the original field notes on which the publication of Davenport & Muncey (1916) was based. A copy was kindly supplied by Dr. Sheldon C. Reed, Dight Institute of Human Genetics, University of Michigan.)

Myrianthopoulos, N. C. & P. T. Rowley (1960). Monozygotic twins concordant for Huntington's chorea. *Neurology (Minneap.)* **10**, 506.

Neel, J. V. & W. J. Schull (1954). *Human Heredity,* p. 49. University of Chicago Press, Chicago.

Neumayer, E. & A. Rett (1966). Ein Choreasippe mit rigider Form. *Wien. Z. Nervenheilk.* **23**, 74.

Oepen, H. (1965). Geschlechtsabhangige Modifikation der Geburtenrate, des Erkrankungs- und des Sterbealters bei Huntingtonscher Chorea. *Homo,* Suppl. 9, p. 296. (Tagung der Deutsche Gesellschaft für Anthropologie, Oct. 1965, Freiburg i. Breslau.)

Oltman, J. E. & S. Friedman (1961). Comments on Huntington's chorea. *Dis. nerv. Syst.* **22**, 313.

Oppenheim, H. (1887). Eine seltene Motilitatsneurose (Chorea hereditaria?). *Berl. klin. Wschr.* **24**, 309.

Ørbeck, A. L. & T. Quelprud (1954). *Setesdalsrykka (chorea progressiva hereditaria).* J. Dybwad, Oslo.

Pache, H. D. (1953). *Mschr. Kinderheilk.* **101**, 504.

Panse, F. (1942). Der Erbchorea. *Sammlung Psychiatrischer und Neurologischer Einzeldarstellung,* Band 18. G. Thieme, Berlin.

Parker, N. (1958). Observations on Huntington's chorea based on a Queensland survey. *Med. J. Aust.* **1**, 351.

Patterson, R. M., B. K. Bagchi & A. Test (1948). The prediction of Huntington's chorea. An electroencephalographic and genetic study. *Amer. J. Psychiat.* **104**, 786.

Pearson, J. S. & M. C. Petersen (1954). Coincidence of Huntington's chorea and multiple neurofibromatosis in two generations. *Amer. J. hum. Genet.* **6**, 344.

Penrose, L. S. & E. M. Watson (1945). A sex-linked tendency in familial diabetes. *Proc. Amer. Diabetes Ass.* **5**, 163.

Peretti, J. (1885). Ueber hereditäre choreatische Bewegungsstorungen. *Berl. klin. Wschr.* **22**, 824.

Petit, H. (1969). La maladie de Huntington. *Rapports 67e Session. Congrès de Psychiatrie et de Neurologie de Langue Francaise,* Brussels. Masson et Cie, Paris.

Pleydell, M. J. (1954). Huntington's chorea in Northamptonshire. *Brit. med. J.* **2**, 1121.

Popenoe, P. & K. Brousseau (1930). Huntington's chorea *J. Hered.* **21**, 113.

Reed, T. E. & J. H. Chandler (1958). Huntington's chorea in Michigan. 1. Demography and genetics. *Amer. J. hum. Genet.* **10**, 201.

Reed, T. E. & J. V. Neel (1959). Huntington's chorea in Michigan. 2. Selection and mutation. *Amer J. hum. Genet.* **11**, 107.

Reisch, O. (1929). Studien an einer Huntington-Sippe. Ein Beitrag zur Symptomatologie verschiedener Stadien der Chorea Huntington. *Arch. Psychiat. Nervenkr.* **86**, 327.

Reisman, L. E. & A. P. Matheny (1969). *Genetics and Counseling in Medical Practice,* p. 54. C. V. Mosby Co., St. Louis.

Riggenbach, M. & A. Werthemann (1933). Untersuchungen bei einer Sippe von Huntington'scher Chorea. *Schweiz. Arch. Neurol. Psychiat.* **31**, 306.

Riggs, C. E. (1901). Three cases of hereditary chorea. *J. nerv. ment. Dis.* **28**, 519.

Saetra, G. (1958). Lund-Huntingtons chorea. En nyoppdaget slekt i ostfold fylke. *T. norske Lægeforen.* **78**, 642.

Saginario, M., V. Corrente, S. Passeri & V. Bagnasco (1967). La variante rigida della corea di Huntington nell'eta' infanto-giovenile. *Sist. nerv.* **5**, 288.

Schlesinger, H. (1892). Ueber einige seltenere Formen der Chorea. I. Chorea chronica hereditaria. II. Chorea chronica congenita. *Z. klin. Med.* **20**, 127, 506.

Schönfelder, T. (1966). Kindliche Chorea Huntington. *Z. Kinderheilk.* **95**, 131.

Schultze, F. (1898). Ueber Poly-Para- und Monoclonien und ihre Beziehungen zur Chorea. *Dtsch. Z. Nervenheilk.* **13**, 409.

Sinkler, W. (1889). Two additional cases of hereditary chorea. *J. nerv. ment. Dis.* **14**, 69.

Sjögren, T. (1935). Vererbungsmedizinische Untersuchungen über Huntingtons Chorea in einer schwedischen Bauernpopulation. *Z. menschl. Vererb.-u. Konstit.-Lehre* **19**, 131.

Smith, C. A. B. (1958). A note on the effects of method of ascertainment on segregation ratios. *Ann. hum. Genet.* **23**, 310.

Sokal, R. R. & F. J. Rohlf (1969). *Biometry.* W. H. Freeman & Co., San Francisco.

Sölder (1895). Chorea chronica. *Neurol. Zbl.* **14**, 1149.

Spillane, J. & R. Phillips (1937). Huntington's chorea in South Wales. *Quart. J. Med.* **6**, 403.

Starr, A. (1967). A disorder of rapid eye movements in Huntington's chorea. *Brain* **90**, 545.

Stevens, D. & M. Parsonage (1969). Mutation in Huntington's chorea. *J. Neurol. Neurosurg. Psychiat.* **32**, 140.

Stone, S. (1932). Chronic progressive chorea (Huntington's disease). *New Engl. J. Med.* **207**, 974.

Stone, T. T. & E. I. Falstein (1939). Genealogical studies in Huntington's chorea. *J. nerv. ment. Dis.* **89**, 795.

Sumner, D. (1962). Amyotrophy in a family with Huntington's chorea. *Wld. Neurol.* **3**, 769.

Tamir, A., J. Whittier & C. Korenyi (1969). Huntington's chorea: a sex difference in psychopathological symptoms. *Dis. nerv. Syst.* **30**, 103.

Tay, C. H. (1970). Huntington's chorea: report of a Chinese family in Singapore. *J. med. Genet.* **7**, 41.

Tsuang, M. (1969). Huntington's chorea in a Chinese family. *J. med. Genet.* **6**, 354.

von Sántha, K. (1931). Zur Pathologie der hereditären Chorea. *Arch. Psychiat. Nervenkr.* **95**, 455.

Wendt, G. G., H. J. Landzettel & I. Unterreiner (1959). Das erkrankungsalter bei der Huntingtonschen Chorea. *Acta genet. (Basel)* **9**, 18.

Wendt, G. G., I. Landzettel & K. Solth (1960). Krankheitsdauer und Lebenserwartung bei der Huntingtonschen Chorea. *Arch. Psychiat. Nervenkr.* **201**, 298.

Wendt, G. G., K. Solth & H. J. Landzettel (1961). Kinderzahl, erkrankungsalter und sterbalter bei der Huntingtonschen Chorea. *Anthrop. Anz.* **24**, 299.

Werner, A. & J. J. Folk (1968). Manifestations of neurotic conflict in Huntington's chorea. A case history. *J. nerv. ment. Dis.* **147**, 141.

Weyrauch, W. (1905). Ueber Chorea chronica progressiva (Huntington'sche Chorea). *Münch. med. Wschr.* **52**, 259.

Worster-Drought, C. & I. M. Allen (1929). Huntington's chorea. *Brit. med. J.* **2**, 1149.

Zacher, O. (1888). Ueber einen Fall von hereditärer Chorea der Erwachsenen. *Neurol. Zbl.* **7**, 34.

Zolliker, A. (1949). Die Chorea Huntington in der Schweiz. *Schweiz. Arch. Neurol. Psychiat.* **64**, 448.

135

Sources of affected sibships

No.	No. of sibships of size														References
	1	2	3	4	5	6	7	8	9	10	11	12	13	14	
1	1														Althaus (1880)
2	1														Arai et al. (1968)
3		1		1											Ballentine (1912)
4		2				1									Barbeau et al. (1964)
5		2	1	1	2										Baron (1950)
6	1		1	1		1									Beaubrun (1963)
7	1														Becker (1938)
8			1		1		1			1					Bell (1934)
9	1	1	3												Bellamy & Green (1961)
10	1			1											Bickford & Ellison (1953)
11	1	2	1												Bittenbender & Quadfasel (1962)
12				1											Bohm (1938)
13	2														Bower (1890)
14	2		1												Briebrecher (1938)
15			1	1		1	1		3	1	1				Brothers (1949)
16			1												Brothers (1964)
17	9	7	1	2	1	4									Brothers & Meadows (1955)
18		1		2			1		1						Buck (1934)
19	1														Byers & Dodge (1967)
20								1							Calkins & van Allen (1967)
21		1													Campbell et al. (1961)
22				1											Chamberlain (1943)
23	2		2	2		1									Chandler et al. (1960)
24											1				Clarke & MacArthur (1924)
25		1													Cronin (1943)
26					1										Curran (1930)
27	3		1		1										Curschmann (1908)
28			1												Dana (1895)
29	1	2													Delmas-Marsalet et al. (1968)
30		1													Dercum (1892)
31	2	1													Dewhurst & Oliver (1970)
32	1			2											D'Ormea (1904)
33		1													Dow (1960)
34					1										El-Garem (1958)
35	2	2	2					1							Entres (1921)
36	3	3	1	1	2			1		1					Entres (1940)
37		1													Evans (1908)
38					1										Ewald (1884)
39			1	1											Facklam (1898)
40	1			1											Finn (1970)
41	2		1												Frank (1937)
42	1														Fraser & Updike (1969)
43	1					2									Frets (1943)
44	1														Freund (1925)
45		1		1	2										Gale & Bennett (1969)
46			1												Gaule (1932)
47	1		1		1										Geratovitsch (1927)
48	1	3		2			1								Gezelle Meerburg (1923)
49	1			1											Goldstein (1913)
50													1		Greppin (1892)
51	1														Gröpl (1968)
52			1	1		1	1								Hamilton (1908)
53	1														Hansotia et al. (1968)
54	1		1		1										Hanssen (1914)
55				1											Harbinson (1880)
56	2		1	1											Hattie (1909)

Appendix I (continued)

No.	1	2	3	4	5	6	7	8	9	10	11	12	13	14	References
57					1										Heathfield (1967)
58		1		1											Hempel (1938)
59		1													Hindringer (1936)
60			1												Hoffmann (1888)
61	1														Hogg (1902)
62	1		1												Huber (1887)
63		2	1												Huet (1889)
64	1		1												Husquinet (1969)
65							1								Jelliffe & White (1917)
66			1												Kloos (1938)
67	1		1												Laane (1951)
68		2		1											Lannois (1888)
69			1		1										Lion & Kahn (1938)
70	1														Lyon (1893)
71	1			1											Lyon (1962)
72		1													Mackay (1904)
73	1			1											Mackenzie-van der Noordaa (1960)
74	2	2	1												Meggendorfer (1923)
75		1		2											Menzies (1892)
76	2														Menzies (1893)
77	1														Mill (1906)
78	3	1	1	1	3	4	4						1		Minski & Guttmann (1938)
79	2				1										Moody (1967)
80			1												Müller-Küppers & Stenzel (1963)
81	74	32	15	13	2	4	2	1		1					Muncey (1964)
82			1												Myrianthopoulos & Rowley (1960)
83	1		1	1		2		1		1					Neel & Schull (1954)
84	1														Neumayer & Rett (1966)
85		1													Oltman & Friedman (1961)
86		1	1												Oppenheim (1887)
87	2				3	2	1								Ørbeck & Quelprud (1954)
88	1	1													Pache (1953)
89	8		1	1		1		1							Panse (1942)
90					1										Parker (1958)
91	4		2												Patterson et al. (1948)
92	2		1				1								Pearson & Petersen (1954)
93			1	1											Peretti (1885)
94	2	2	2		1										Petit (1969)
95	4	2	3	1		1		1							Pleydell (1954)
96			2												Popenoe & Brousseau (1930)
97	1	1					1		1						Reisch (1929)
98	1	1	2												Reisman & Matheny (1969)
99	2		1												Riggenbach & Werthemann (1933)
100				1											Riggs (1901)
101						1									Saetra (1958)
102		1	1												Saginario et al. (1967)
103				1											Schlesinger (1892)
104		1	1	1		2		1							Schönfelder (1966)
105		1													Schultze (1898)
106		2													Sinkler (1889)
107	1		1	1	2		1								Sjögren (1935)
108							1								Sölder (1895)
109		2					1								Spillane & Phillips (1937)
110	2	1	1												Starr (1967)
111			1												Stevens & Parsonage (1969)
112		4	2						1	1					Stone (1932)
113	1	2	3												Stone & Falstein (1939)
114			1												Sumner (1962)

137

No.	No. of sibships of size														References
	1	2	3	4	5	6	7	8	9	10	11	12	13	14	
115				1											Tay (1970)
116			1			1									Tsuang (1969)
117			1												Von Sántha (1931)
118	1														Werner & Folk (1968)
119		1													Weyrauch (1905)
120		1													Worster-Drought & Allen (1929)
121			1												Zacher (1888)
122	2	1	2										1		Zolliker (1949)

Appendix II

Number of sibships in relation to location and decade of publication of data

Location	1860–9	1870–9	1880–9	1890–9	1900–9	1910–9	1920–9	1930–9	1940–9	1950–9	1960–9	1970–9	Total
U.S.A.	1		2	4	6	147		18	7	11	35	2	233
Germany			10	6	6	2	20	13	24	2	8		91
Great Britain			1	5	2		1	26		14	6	3	58
Australia					1				9	25	5		40
France			6							6	10		22
Norway						3				11			14
Canada					4		1	5			3		13
The Netherlands							7		3		2		12
Switzerland								4	6				10
Sweden								6					6
Italy					3						2		5
West Indies											4		4
Belgium											2		2
Formosa											2		2
Austria											2		2
Egypt											1		1
Japan										1			1
New Zealand									1				1
Singapore												1	1
Total	1		19	15	22	152	29	72	50	70	81	6	517

139

The Metabolism of Low Density Lipoprotein in Familial Type II Hyperlipoproteinemia

Terry Langer, Warren Strober, and Robert I. Levy

INTRODUCTION

Familial type II hyperlipoproteinemia is a lipid transport disorder transmitted as an autosomal dominant and characterized by a marked elevation in the concentration of plasma low density (S_f 0–12, density $1.019 - 1.063$) beta lipoprotein (LDL),[1] hypercholesterolemia, xanthomatosis, and premature coronary atherosclerosis (2).

The primary metabolic abnormalities responsible for the hyperlipoproteinemia and hypercholesterolemia in type II patients have not been elucidated. One possibility is that the abnormality in type II hyperlipoproteinemia involves a defect in the metabolism of LDL and more specifically that of the protein moiety of LDL rather than one of its lipid constituents (3). To study this question we have performed, and now report on, metabolic studies

This work was presented in part at the 61st Annual Meeting of the American Society for Clinical Investigation, Atlantic City, N. J., May 1969

[1] *Abbreviations used in this paper:* FCR, fractional catabolic rate; LDL, low density lipoprotein; P, plasma; U, urinary.

with purified, radioiodinated plasma LDL in normal individuals and patients with type II hyperlipoproteinemia.

METHODS

Patients

Normal patients. 10 normal patients (6 men and 4 women) were studied. Clinical data for these individuals are summarized in Table I. Each patient had normal thyroid, hepatic, and renal function and normal glucose tolerance tests. None of the normal patients had a family history of hyperlipoproteinemia.

Type II patients. 10 patients with heterozygous familial type II hyperlipoproteinemia were studied (6 men and 4 women). Clinical data for these patients are summarized in Table II. The clinical diagnosis was established in all 10 by: (*a*) the presence of marked elevations of plasma LDL in the absence of clinical or chemical evidence of other disorders associated with secondary hyperbetalipoproteinemia (i.e., hypothyroidism, hepatic disease, nephrotic syndrome, or dysglobulinemia) (3), (*b*) the presence of at least one similarly affected first degree relative, and (*c*) the presence of characteristic tendon xanthomata.

All patients were studied on the metabolic wards of the Clinical Center of the National Heart and Lung Institute and were fed a balanced diet containing < 300 mg of cholesterol/day and a ratio of polyunsaturated to saturated fat of approximately 2.5/1 with 40% of the calories derived from fat, 40% from carbohydrate, and 20% from protein. Body weight, total plasma cholesterol, triglyceride, and LDL-cholesterol concentrations were measured serially throughout each study period and remained constant. None of the patients or volunteers were taking medications during the period of study.

Preparation of LDL

LDL was prepared from plasma of type II patients and normals. Blood (150 ml) was collected in sterile, pyrogen-free plastic bags containing a 1% solution of the disodium salt of ethylenediaminetetraacetic acid (EDTA) (15 ml). The plasma was immediately separated by centrifugation at 4°C and its density adjusted to 1.019 g/ml by the addition of a solution of NaCl-KBr of density 1.085 g/ml. The plasma was then subjected to preparative ultracentrifugation for 12 hr at 40,000 rpm in a Spinco No. 40 rotor (Beckman Instruments, Inc., Fullerton, Calif.) after which the d < 1.019 g/ml (i.e., $S_f > 12$) supernate was removed by tube slicing. The infranate was then adjusted to a density of 1.063 g/ml by the addition of NaCl-KBr solution of density 1.35 g/ml and subjected to further ultracentrifugation for 12 hr in a Spinco No. 65 rotor at 65,000 rpm after which the supernate containing lipoprotein of density range 1.019–1.063 g/ml was isolated. This material was then washed and concentrated by a final ultracentrifugation after carefully overlayering with NaCl-KBr solution of density

TABLE I
Clinical Data, Normals*

Initials	Sex	Age	Weight	Plasma cholesterol	LDL cholesterol	Plasma glycerides
		yr	kg	mg/ 100 ml	mg/ 100 ml	mg/ 100 ml
A. R.	F	42	60.1	167	116	72
J. R.	F	24	47.0	189	151	134
N. E.	F	21	52.9	134	84	62
B. S.	F	21	67.8	172	114	52
S. G.	M	24	75.2	114	82	66
A. A.	M	21	57.5	153	119	81
B. S.	M	22	64.6	147	108	89
E. S.	M	26	60.0	142	100	51
B. V. C.	M	22	70.6	142	89	47
B. B.	M	22	72.7	153	88	81

* Lipid values are those obtained after 2 wk on a low cholesterol, high polyunsaturated/saturated ratio diet (see text).

TABLE II
Clinical Data, Type II Patients*

Initials	Sex	Age	Weight	Plasma cholesterol	LDL cholesterol	Plasma glycerides
		yr	kg	mg/ 100 ml	mg/ 100 ml	mg/ 100 ml
B. C.	F	34	54.6	359	308	136
M. B.	F	62	61.1	324	249	135
T. G.	F	27	62.5	238	196	73
A. B.	F	39	48.5	355	271	106
H. J.	M	36	72.4	373	310	134
J. B.	M	32	57.6	254	190	85
G. H.	M	35	83.7	365	273	204
H. K.	M	49	55.5	341	304	162
A. L.	M	48	70.2	287	236	139
S. T.	M	40	75.7	300	204	96

* Lipid values are those obtained after 2 wk on a low cholesterol, high polyunsaturated/saturated ratio diet (see text).

1.063 g/ml. As a final purification step, concentrated LDL was dialyzed overnight against 0.15 M NaCl containing 0.1% EDTA, pH 7.4, in order to remove KBr and return the preparation to plasma density (1.006 g/ml).

Each preparation of LDL used in turnover studies was demonstrated to be free of contaminating lipoproteins by

142

immunoelectrophoresis in agarose gel employing specific antisera prepared against high density (alpha), low density (beta) lipoproteins, and very low density lipoprotein apoproteins (4). In addition, no other contaminating serum proteins were found using antisera reacting with albumin, gamma globulin, and whole human serum (4).

Canine LDL was prepared in a similar fashion, except that the lipoprotein of d = 1.019 − 1.050 was isolated to minimize contamination with HDL which, in the dog, is present in considerably greater amounts than LDL. In addition, tests of lipoprotein purity were conducted using antisera specific for canine plasma proteins and lipoproteins.

Radioiodination

Radiolabeling of LDL was carried out using a modification of the iodine monochloride method of McFarlane (5). Purified LDL protein (10–40 mg) in a volume of 1.0–1.5 ml was labeled with carrier-free ^{125}I at 4°C in 1.0 M glycine-NaOH buffer, pH 10. In vitro studies revealed that the efficiency of iodination, i.e. the fraction of the radioiodine in the reaction mixture which is bound to LDL, was maximal at pH 9.0–10.0, but the proportion of the label which was bound to lipid (rather than protein) was minimal at the higher pH (Fig. 1). The efficiency of iodination at pH 10 was 10–25% and this resulted in the attachment of approximately 0.5 atoms of iodine to each LDL molecule (assuming a molecular weight for LDL of 2×10^6 (6, 7) of which 25% by weight is protein [8]).

Unbound iodine was removed by dialysis vs. 0.15 M NaCl, 0.1% EDTA, pH 7.4. After dialysis the ^{125}I-LDL preparations all contained less than 1% free ^{125}I as determined by

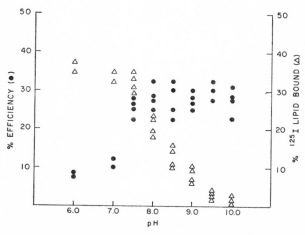

FIGURE 1 Effect of pH of iodination medium on efficiency of iodination (●) and percentage of ^{125}I bound to the lipid moiety of LDL (△).

143

precipitation with 10% trichloroacetic acid (TCA) and 5% phosphotungstic acid in the presence of carrier albumin, cold LDL, or plasma.

The extent of lipid labeling was determined by extraction of labeled LDL with a 2:1 chloroform:methanol solvent (9). It was found that the fraction of radioiodine bound to lipid was related to the overall efficiency of the labeling procedure and to the pH. Lipid labeling was minimal at higher pH: the mean fraction of lipid extractable lipoprotein-bound radioiodine was 2.4% (range 1.8–3.4%) at pH 10. The distribution of lipid-bound radioactivity among the various lipid constituents of LDL was determined by thin-layer chromatography of chloroform-methanol extracts. The lipid extracts were evaporated to dryness under nitrogen, redissolved with small amounts of $CHCl_3$–CH_3OH solvent, applied to thin-layer chromatographic plates, and run in polar (chloroform-ethanol-water: : 195:75:12) and nonpolar (petroleum ether: ethyl ether: glacial acetic acid: : 90:10:1) solvent systems along with appropriate standards (10). The plates were dried, stained with anisaldehyde or iodine vapor, and the bands sequentially scraped and counted. The major portion of lipid-bound ^{125}I was associated with phospholipids, especially lecithin, with smaller amounts associated with free cholesterol, cholesterol ester, and glyceride.

The iodination procedure did not affect the electrophoretic behavior or immunologic reactivity of the LDL as demonstrated by simultaneous agarose-gel immunoelectrophoresis (4) and paper electrophoresis (11) of unlabeled and radiolabeled LDL. Furthermore, the paper electrophoretograms were scanned to localize small amounts of labeled proteins which did not migrate with LDL; in all cases, > 95% of the radioactivity was localized to the beta₂ globulin band characteristic of native LDL.

Iodination did not affect the flotation characteristics of LDL. The ^{125}I-LDL was mixed with human plasma from a normal fasting individual and ultracentrifuged at densities 1.006, 1.019, 1.063, and 1.21 g/ml (after addition of appropriate quantities of NaCl-KBr solution and solid KBr) to determine if gross alterations in flotation were produced by radioiodination. These studies demonstrated that > 98% of the radioactivity could be recovered between densities 1.019 and 1.063 g/ml.

Preparation of ^{125}I-LDL for in vivo studies

Immediately after removal of unbound ^{125}I by dialysis, sterile human albumin was added to the ^{125}I-LDL preparations to minimize damage due to self-radiation. The preparation was then passed through a 0.45 mμ Millipore filter (Millipore Corp., Bedford, Mass.) and tested for sterility and pyrogenicity before in vivo studies. Final dilutions of each preparation were made with buffered saline containing 0.1% EDTA; such dilutions contained 35 mg/ml of albumin and 10 μCi/ml of ^{125}I-LDL. The ^{125}I-LDL was usually considered ready for reinjection approximately 96 hr after the original plasma sample was obtained.

Study protocol

Metabolic studies in dogs. Mongrel dogs weighing approximately 20 kg were placed in metabolic cages with free access to food and water containing sodium iodide. To obtain ^{125}I-LDL plasma decay curves, 25–50 μCi of ^{125}I-LDL prepared as described above were administered intravenously to fasting animals and serial blood samples obtained from the opposite foreleg 10 min after injection and daily for 7–10 days thereafter. A series of "screening" experiments were conducted to detect the presence of denatured, rapidly degradable protein in the ^{125}I-LDL preparations. In these experiments a first set of dogs was injected with 1–2 mCi of freshly prepared ^{125}I-LDL and then plasmapheresed approximately 24 hr later. During this period these animals clear and degrade any denatured material which is present in the preparation. The residual "biologically screened" ^{125}I-LDL contained in the 24 hr plasma sample is then reinjected into a second set of dogs and plasma samples collected as in the usual study.

Metabolic studies in humans. Fasting, supine patients and normals were administered 25–50 μCi of ^{125}I-LDL (approximately 1–2 mg of LDL apoprotein) intravenously from a calibrated syringe via a continuous saline infusion. Subsequently, 10-ml blood samples were collected in glass tubes containing EDTA at 10 min ("zero time"), 1, 4, 8, 12, 24, 36, 48, 60, and 72 hr and then daily for 14 days. The plasma was immediately separated at 4°C and portions removed for counting and total cholesterol determinations. 40-ml fasting samples were obtained on days 1, 3, 7, 10, and 14 and subjected to complete lipoprotein quantification (3). 24 hr urine specimens were collected in glass jars containing small amounts of KI, NaHSO₃, and NaOH to minimize volatilization of ^{125}I or its adsorption to glass. The patients received 1.0 g of KI daily by mouth in divided doses for 3 days before and throughout each study to inhibit uptake of radioiodine by the thyroid. Informed consent was obtained from each patient and normal volunteer.

Sample analysis

2-ml portions of the daily plasma samples and 5-ml portions from the 24-hr urine collections were counted along with appropriate standards in an automatic gamma-ray, well-type scintillation counter. In early studies, every plasma sample was precipitated with 10% TCA to determine if nonprotein-bound ^{125}I accounted for a significant proportion of radioactivity. In every case it was found that < 3% of the radioactivity consisted of nonprotein-bound iodide; hence in later studies this procedure was discontinued and it was assumed that total plasma radioactivity represented protein-bound ^{125}I.

Each plasma sample was analyzed for total cholesterol content. In addition, larger samples were obtained during each study for a more complete lipid analysis including determination of triglycerides, high density, low density, and very low density lipoprotein cholesterol concentration using methods previously described (3). In these studies, LDL of density 1.019–1.063 g/ml was isolated separately for

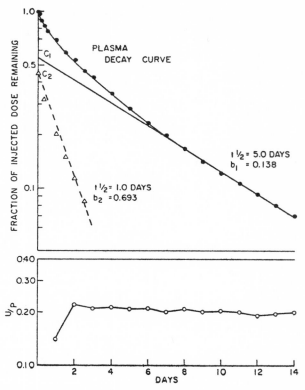

FIGURE 2 *Upper panel:* Typical LDL plasma decay curve with exponentials. First exponential is the terminal (linear) portion of decay curve extrapolated to zero time. Second exponential is the plot of values obtained from subtracting first exponential from original decay curve. *Lower panel:* Metabolic clearance values (U/P values) of LDL plotted for each day of a typical study. Initial value is low because of delay in iodide excretion. Constancy of subsequent values indicates metabolic homogeneity of labeled LDL.

lipid analysis. Portions of the larger samples were also subjected to ultracentrifugation at densities 1.006, 1.019, 1.063, and 1.21 g/ml to determine the flotation characteristics of the circulating ^{125}I-LDL. Finally, a portion of the original purified, unlabeled LDL isolated from each subject was also analyzed for protein (12), total cholesterol (13), triglyceride (14), and phospholipid (15).

Data analysis

The metabolic parameters governing the turnover of LDL were calculated by methods described by Matthews (16) and by Nosslin (17) for the analysis of plasma decay curves (Fig. 2, upper panel).

146

The fractional catabolic rate (FCR) (the fraction of the intravascular LDL pool catabolized per day) was calculated using the expression: Fractional catabolic rate $= 1/(C_1/b_1 + C_2/b_2)$, where C_n and b_n are the y intercepts and slopes of the plasma radioactivity decay curve and its peeled exponentials (see reference 16). The distribution of LDL between the intravascular and extravascular compartments was calculated using the expression:

$$\% \text{ intravascular} = \left[\frac{C_1}{b_1} + \frac{C_2}{b_2}\right]^2 \bigg/ \frac{C_1}{(b_1)^2} + \frac{C_2}{(b_2)^2}.$$

The plasma volume was calculated by isotopic dilution using the 10 min plasma sample on the assumption that during this interval the distribution of ^{125}I-LDL was uniform and that insignificant amounts of labeled lipoprotein were catabolized or entered the extravascular compartment. The total intravascular LDL-cholesterol pool was computed from the product of the LDL-cholesterol concentration (the mean of five determinations of LDL-cholesterol concentration during each study) and the plasma volume. The intravascular LDL-apoprotein pool was then calculated from the product of the LDL-cholesterol pool and the ratio of LDL-apoprotein/LDL-cholesterol which was measured for each subject. (This ratio was approximately 0.6).

The steady-state synthetic rate (or absolute catabolic rate) was then calculated as follows: synthetic rate $=$ FCR $\times$ intravascular LDL-apoprotein. The synthetic rate was expressed as milligrams of apoprotein synthesized per day normalized for body weight (milligrams/kilogram per day).

In addition to the method described above for the calculation of the fractional catabolic rate (which relies solely on the plasma decay curve) an independent estimate of the FCR was obtained from the daily urinary radioactivity excretion using the metabolic clearance method of Berson and Yalow (18). With this method, the clearance of ^{125}I-LDL is calculated for each day of the study from the ratio of total urinary radioactivity excreted in each 24 hr period to the mean plasma radioactivity during that interval (Fig. 2, lower plane). This U/P ratio is an accurate estimate of the fractional catabolic rate provided the rate of iodide excretion is rapid compared to rate of LDL breakdown.

RESULTS

Animal studies

The mean fractional catabolic rate (± 1 SD) of unscreened human ^{125}I-LDL obtained in eight dogs using four different protein preparations was 0.0338 ± 0.0030 of the intravascular pool/hr (0.810 ± 0.070/day); this corresponded to a biological half-life of 26.6 ± 1.7 hr. The FCR and biological half-life of four additional preparations of human ^{125}I-LDL which had first been screened for 18–24 hr in dogs was 0.0326 ± 0.0019/hr (0.781 ± 0.045/day) corresponding to a biological half-life of

147

TABLE III
Metabolic Parameters, Normals

Initials	Plasma volume	Plasma APO-LDL	Intra-vascular*	Fractional catabolic rate (fraction of IV pool/day)		Biological half-life (t‡)	Synthetic rate	
	ml	mg/ 100 ml	%	A‡	B§	days	mg/day	mg/kg per day
A. R.	2927	70	65.2	0.452	0.365	3.58	926	15.4
J. R.	2250	91	66.4	0.418	0.400	3.33	856	18.2
N. E.	2807	51	64.4	0.528	0.486	3.00	756	14.3
B. S.	2616	80	69.2	0.398	0.385	3.00	1041	15.3
S. G.	3515	49	75.0	0.633	0.653	2.25	1090	14.5
A. A.	2737	72	69.8	0.385	0.364	3.25	759	13.2
B. S.	3102	65	66.4	0.445	0.370	3.25	897	13.9
E. S.	2780	60	70.0	0.455	0.423	3.00	759	12.5
B. V. C.	3410	62	75.3	0.393	0.405	3.10	841	12.0
B. B.	3432	62	62.6	0.511	0.492	3.17	1087	15.0

* Per cent of APO-LDL pool in intravascular compartment.

‡ Calculated from serum decay curve by method of Matthews‾ (16); see text.

§ Calculated from U/P ratios; see text.

27.0±0.8 days; these values were not significantly different from the unscreened preparations ($P > 0.4$) and there was therefore no evidence for the presence of rapidly degradable protein in the ^{125}I-LDL preparations. It was of interest that ^{125}I-LDL injected into a dog 2 wk after labeling contained a considerable amount of rapidly degradable material; in this case the plasma decay curve showed a rapid early decline followed by a normal terminal slope. This observation suggests that radioactive LDL must be used promptly after purification and labeling.

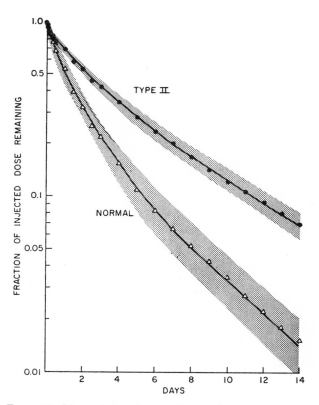

FIGURE 3 Mean plasma decay (die-away) curves for normal individuals ($\triangle$) and patients with type II hyperlipoproteinemia ($\bullet$). Shaded areas indicate 1 SD on either side of mean. Since the fractional catabolic rate is equal to the reciprocal of the areas under these curves, it is clear that type II patients have a lower fractional catabolic rate than normal individuals.

149

Identical plasma decay curves were observed when ^{125}I-LDL obtained from normal individuals and patients with type II hyperlipoproteinemia were injected into dogs, suggesting that there are no major structural differences in the LDL molecules from these two sources. On the other hand, canine LDL demonstrated a considerably slower rate of degradation than LDL from human sources. In this case the FCR was 0.0262 of the intravascular pool/hr (0.628/day) and the biological half-life was 38.5 hr.

Throughout each study in the dogs, greater than 95% of the plasma radioactivity could be reisolated between the densities 1.019 and 1.063 g/ml and less than 1% of the radioactivity was found in the density 1.21 g/ml infranate, indicating that, in the dog, the labeled LDL circulates as an intact lipoprotein and does not associate with or become converted to lipoproteins of other densities.

Human studies

LDL metabolism in normal subjects (Table III) (Figs. 3 and 4). In 10 normal individuals the mean FCR of autologous LDL was 0.462±0.077 of the intravascular pool/day (range 0.385 — 0.633/day) and the mean biological half-life was 3.08±0.35 days (range 2.25 — 3.58 days). The mean synthetic rate of LDL apoprotein was 14.43±1.75 mg/kg per day (range 12.0–18.2 mg/kg per day) or 901.2±132.2 mg/day (range: 756–1090 mg/day).The mean percentage of the total exchangeable LDL confined to the intravascular compartment was 68.4±4.3% (range 62.6–75.0%).

LDL metabolism in subjects with familial type II hyperlipoproteinemia (Table IV) (Figs. 3 and 4). In 10 patients with type II hyperlipoproteinemia the mean FCR of autologous LDL was 0.237±0.044 of the intravascular pool/day (range: 0.205 — 0.352 of the intravascular pool/day) and the mean biological half-life was 4.68±0.044 days (range: 3.80–5.17 days); both of these parameters are significantly different from normal ($P <$ 0.001). The mean synthetic rate of LDL-apoprotein was 15.01±1.71 mg/kg per day (range: 12.2 — 17.5 mg/kg per day) or 955.0±147.5 mg/day (range: 769–1255 mg/day) and 73.3±5.2% (65.0–83.2%) of the total exchangeable LDL was in the intravascular space. The synthetic rate of LDL in type II patients was not significantly different from normal ($P >$ 0.4), nor was the distribution of LDL among the body spaces ($P >$ 0.05).

U/P ratios. In all studies the fractional catabolic

150

TABLE IV
Metabolic Parameters, Type II Patients

Initials	Plasma volume	Plasma APO-LDL	Intra-vascular*	Fractional cata-bolic rate		Biological half-life ($t_\frac{1}{2}$)	Synthetic rate	
	ml	*mg/ 100 ml*	%	A‡	B§	*days*	*mg/day*	*mg/kg per day*
				fraction of IV pool/day				
B. C.	2234	185	71.6	0.211	0.207	5.17	872	16.0
M. B.	2500	149	74.1	0.221	0.221	4.90	823	13.5
T. G.	2694	118	65.0	0.352	0.348	3.80	1038	16.6
A. B.	1940	163	74.2	0.257	0.241	4.00	812	16.7
H. J.	2681	186	72.3	0.217	0.215	5.00	1082	15.0
J. B.	2835	114	71.9	0.238	0.238	4.70	769	13.3
G. H.	3430	164	83.2	0.223	0.236	4.67	1255	15.0
H. K.	2601	182	76.5	0.205	0.208	4.93	970	17.5
S. T.	3147	122	66.5	0.241	0.233	4.83	925	12.2
A. L.	3414	142	77.4	0.207	0.199	4.83	1004	14.3

* Per cent of APO-LDL pool in intravascular compartment.
‡ Calculated from serum decay curve by the method of Matthews (16); see text.
§ Calculated from U/P ratios; see text.

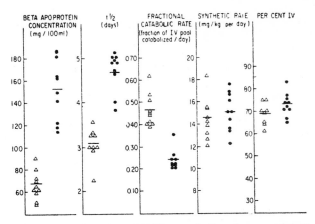

FIGURE 4 Parameters of LDL metabolism in normal individuals (△) and patients with type II hyperlipoproteinemia (●). Fractional catabolic rate of LDL is greatly reduced in the patient group (3rd panel) whereas synthetic rate is normal (4th panel). Horizontal bars represent mean values.

rate obtained from the mean U/P ratio was in close agreement with the FCR calculated from the plasma decay curve (Tables III and IV). The U/P ratio for the 1st day of each turnover study was always considerably lower than for succeeding days and this value was excluded from the calculations. This finding was attributed to the normal delay in iodide excretion after ^{125}I-LDL catabolism. The U/P ratio for the remainder of each study was constant except for a few cases within the normal group when this parameter decreased slightly in the last few days of the study at a time when the total remaining plasma radioactivity was considerably less than 3% of the injected dose. This gradual decline in the U/P ratio was not seen in any study involving patients with type II hyperlipoproteinemia including one study which was continued for an additional 7 days. It was concluded from the constancy of the U/P ratio that the ^{125}I-LDL molecules in each preparation had uniform metabolic behavior and that no significant amounts of rapidly degradable protein were present.

Flotation of plasma ^{125}I-LDL. Throughout each study, greater than 95% of the circulating radioactivity was recovered by ultracentrifugation between densities 1.019 and 1.063 g/ml, with less than 1% in the 1.21 g/ml infranate. These data confirmed the in vitro and animal studies and provided evidence that LDL-apoprotein is not converted or incorporation into lipoproteins of other density classes, nor does it circulate in significant amounts as the free apoprotein at a density greater than 1.21 g/ml.

The metabolism of isologous ^{125}*I-LDL in patients with type II hyperlipoproteinemia.* To determine if

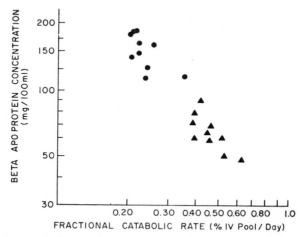

FIGURE 5 Relationships between beta apoprotein concentration (mg/100 ml) and LDL fractional catabolic rate (% intravascular [IV] pool/day) in normal individuals (△) and patients with type II hyperlipoproteinemia (●).

the differences in the catabolism of LDL in normal individuals and patients with type II hyperlipoproteinemia resulted from inherent differences in the circulating LDL molecules, the turnover of ^{125}I-LDL which had been isolated from a normal individual was studied in three subjects with type II disease who had previously received autologous ^{125}I-LDL. No differences in metabolic behavior were noted between the autologous and isologous proteins. The FCR, biological half-life, and U/P ratios were virtually identical in each paired study.

DISCUSSION

In the present investigation, radioiodinated, purified low density lipoprotein (d = 1.019 − 1.063 g/ml) was used to determine the behavior of LDL in normal individuals and patients with heterozygous familial type II hyperlipoproteinemia.

Studies of ^{125}*I-LDL turnover in normal individuals.* The metabolic parameters of LDL apoprotein in normal individuals obtained with iodinated preparations used in these studies are comparable to the values reported by Volwiler et al. (19) using biosynthetically labeled ^{35}S-LDL and by Gitlin et al. (20), Walton et al. (21, 22), Scott and Winterbourn (23), and Hurly and Scott (24), using radioiodinated LDL. We did not observe a difference in LDL metabolism between men and women as reported by others (23, 24).

LDL has several singular metabolic features when compared with other plasma proteins. To begin with, although LDL is similar to other large serum proteins such as IgM and fibrinogen with regard to its distribution among the body compartments, the fractional catabolic rate of LDL is significantly greater than these proteins (25, 26). This suggests that LDL may be acted upon by a unique catabolic mechanism not shared by other proteins, or more likely, that LDL is subject to a specific degradation mechanism which acts in addition to a more generalized catabolic mechanism. This hypothesis is supported by studies which indicate that LDL clearance and degradation are linked to bile acid and cholesterol metabolism and transport. In this regard, we have shown that the administration of cholestyramine results in an increase in the fractional catabolic rate of LDL of type II patients (27). Since the action of cholestyramine is limited to the intraluminal binding of bile salts in the gastrointestinal tract, the effect of this perturbation on LDL metabolism would be mediated through changes in bile acid and/or cholesterol metabolism presumably occurring in the liver.

Another unusual attribute of LDL metabolism is the observation that, to a greater extent than other plasma proteins, the physiologic control of LDL concentration appears to be mediated via changes in catabolic rates rather than by alterations in synthetic rates (28). Thus, the normal patient with the lowest LDL concentration had the highest fractional catabolic rate and, in general, the plasma LDL concentration was inversely proportional to the fractional catabolic rate (Fig. 5). In contrast, the synthetic rate was not correlated with plasma LDL levels and was relatively constant. These observations are consonant with the finding that changes in dietary cholesterol and saturated fatty acid content exert their effect on LDL concentration in normal patients by changing the fractional catabolic rate of LDL whereas synthetic rates remain unchanged (27). A similar relationship between LDL

154

concentration and fractional catabolic rate is observed in patients with type II hyperlipoproteinemia, but in this case the entire range of LDL concentrations is shifted to a higher level (Fig. 5).

Studies of ^{125}I-LDL metabolism in patients with type II hyperlipoproteinemia. Patients with type II hyperlipoproteinemia had normal synthetic rates for LDL and a normal distribution of the lipoprotein in the body compartments. However, all patients demonstrated a striking decrease in the fractional catabolic rate of LDL which in each case was sufficient to account for the elevation in plasma LDL concentration. Since we could detect no differences in the metabolic behavior of autologous and isologous LDL from normal individuals when injected into patients with type II disease or into dogs, it is apparent that this defect in LDL metabolism is not intrinsic to the LDL molecule itself but instead resides in the catabolic mechanisms for LDL in these hyperlipoproteinemic patients. The abnormality in LDL catabolism in type II patients can therefore be visualized as a resetting of the LDL catabolic mechanism so that it operates at a lower range of fractional catabolic rates at the expense of an expanded plasma LDL pool.

Our results differ from previous studies of the behavior of LDL in hyperlipoproteinemic individuals. Walton et al. (21) and Scott and Hurley (29) found that the biological half-life and the fractional catabolic rate of LDL in type II patients were not significantly different from normal and concluded that excessive LDL synthesis was responsible for the hyperlipoproteinemia. It is likely from the data presented by these authors that many of these individuals did not have type II hyperlipoproteinemia. Furthermore it is possible that some of their patients represent an isolate within the broad definition of familial type II hyperlipoproteinemia who synthesize excessive amounts of LDL and who differ from our type II patients who display defective catabolism of LDL.

The finding of a decreased fractional catabolic rate in patients with type II hyperlipoproteinemia was unexpected since pathologic elevations in plasma protein concentration are usually due primarily to changes in the rate of protein synthesis. We therefore considered the possibility that the observed depression of FCR was a secondary metabolic phenomenon resulting from a primary change in synthetic rate or in the pool size

155

of LDL. This hypothesis is made unlikely by the following considerations. In the first place, one cannot postulate that increased LDL synthesis led to an expanded LDL pool since the measured synthetic rates in hyperlipoproteinemic individuals are normal. In addition, it would be more reasonable to expect that the expansion of the LDL pool would be followed by a homeostatic increase in fractional catabolic rate so as to reestablish the original plasma protein concentration; this response is typical of the metabolic behavior of plasma IgG and to a lesser extent albumin when the pool sizes of these proteins are altered (30). In the second place, recent observations suggest that the fractional catabolic rate of LDL is independent of pool size. Studies from our laboratory have demonstrated that the reduction of LDL synthesis and decrease in the plasma pool of LDL in normal and hyperlipoproteinemic subjects induced by nicotinic acid are not accompanied by changes in the fractional catabolic rate (31). In addition, the fractional catabolic rate of LDL was normal in three individuals with familial hypobetalipoproteinemia who had synthetic rates and concentrations of LDL which were less than one-third of normal (32). Finally, Lees, and Ahrens (33) have demonstrated that the rate of disappearance of infused LDL was constant in an individual with abetalipoproteinemia, despite a constantly changing LDL pool size as LDL was removed from the plasma. For these various reasons, the observed decreased fractional catabolic rate in type II patients is not likely to be secondary to a primary change in LDL synthetic rate or pool size.

The metabolic defect in type II hyperlipoproteinemia. We have concluded that a decreased fractional catabolic rate of LDL is responsible for the hyperlipoproteinemia in patients with type II disease but the mechanism underlying this metabolic abnormality remains unclear. The metabolic defect responsible for the abnormal catabolism of LDL in type II hyperlipoproteinemia could be related to a primary disturbance in the metabolism of the intact lipoprotein or the LDL apoprotein, or it could be the consequence of a more fundamental abnormality in the metabolism of one of the lipid moieties of LDL.

As to the latter possibility, efforts to find a primary lipid abnormality have focused on the supposition that cholesterol synthesis was increased in type II hyperlipoproteinemia. In this regard, no consistent abnormality in the synthesis of cholesterol has been found in individuals with type II disease studied either by the incorporation of acetate-^{14}C into cholesterol, by the analysis of cholesterol-^{14}C decay curves and by fecal sterol balance techniques (34–38). Indeed, recent studies by Goodman and Noble (37) have shown that both normal and hypercholesterolemic individuals synthesize and degrade equal amounts of cholesterol daily.

Whereas cholesterol synthetic rates may be normal, the fractional rate of cholesterol degradation may be depressed in type II patients. Nestel, Whyte, and Goodman (39), using the two-pool model for cholesterol metabolism of Goodman and Noble, have shown that the plasma cholesterol concentration was not related to the production rate or the amount of cholesterol in the two exchangeable pools in normal and hyperlipidemic individuals. However, they determined that the clearance of plasma cholesterol, expressed as a fraction of the total mass of cholesterol in the plasma, is depressed in hypercholesterolemic patients. This observation on cholesterol metabolism appears to parallel our own regarding LDL metabolism and could be the more fundamental abnormality. Thus, it may be argued that a defect in the transport and/or degradation of cholesterol (either cholesterol bound to circulating LDL or cholesterol in some other body compartment) is responsible for the decreased catabolism of plasma LDL in type II patients. Just as reasonably, however, a defect in plasma LDL catabolism may be primary to a similar defect in cholesterol metabolism. In point of fact, the available data do not allow any conclusion as to which phenomenon is cause and which is effect. In any case, our questions concerning the abnormality in type II hyperbetalipoproteinemia have been focused and we now ask: what is the basis of the defect in LDL catabolism in this disease?

REFERENCES

1. Langer, T., W. Strober, and R. I. Levy. 1969. Familial type II hyperlipoproteinemia: a defect of beta lipoprotein apoprotein catabolism? *J. Clin. Invest.* **48:** 49a. (Abstr.)
2. Fredrickson, D. S., and R. I. Levy. 1972. Familial hyperlipoproteinemia. *In* The Metabolic Basis of Inherited Disease. J. B. Stanberry, J. B. Wyngaarden, and D. S. Fredrickson, editors. McGraw-Hill Book Company, Inc., New York. 3rd edition. 545.

3. Fredrickson, D. S., R. I. Levy, and R. S. Lees. 1967. Fat transport in lipoproteins—an integrated approach to mechanisms and disorders. *N. Engl. J. Med.* **276**: 32, 94, 148, 215, and 273.

4. Levy, R. I., R. S. Lees, and D. S. Fredrickson. 1966. The nature of pre-beta (very low density) lipoproteins. *J. Clin. Invest.* **45**: 63.

5. McFarlane, A. S. 1958. Efficient trace-labelling of proteins with iodine. *Nature (London).* **182**: 53.

6. Adams, G. H., and V. N. Schumaker. 1968. Rapid molecular weight estimates for low-density lipoproteins. *Anal. Biochem.* **29**: 117.

7. Lindgren, F. T., L. C. Jensen, R. D. Wills, and N. K. Freeman. 1969. Flotation rates, molecular weights and hydrated densities of the low-density lipoproteins. *Lipids.* **4**: 337.

8. Bragdon, J. H.. R. J. Havel, and E. Boyle. 1956. Human serum lipoproteins. I. Chemical composition of four fractions. *J. Lab. Clin. Med.* **48**: 36.

9. Sperry, W. M., and F. C. Brand. 1955. The determination of total lipides in blood serum. *J. Biol. Chem.* **213**: 69.

10. Kwiterovich, F. O., Jr., H. R. Sloan, and D. S. Fredrickson. 1970. Glycolipids and other lipid constituents of normal human liver. *J. Lipid Res.* **11**: 322.

11. Lees, R. S., and F. T. Hatch. 1963. Sharper separation of lipoprotein species by paper electrophoresis in albumin-containing buffer. *J. Lab. Clin. Med.* **61**: 518.

12. Lowry, D. H., N. J. Rosebrough, A. C. Fall, and R. J. Randall. 1951. Protein measurements with Folin phenol reagent. *J. Biol. Chem.* **193**: 265.

13. Total cholesterol procedure N-24b. 1964. *In* Auto-Analyzer Manual. Technicon Co., Inc., Tarrytown, N. Y.

14. Kessler, G., and H. Lederer. 1965. Fluorometric measurement of triglycerides. *In* Automation in Analytical Chemistry. L. T. Skeggs, Jr., editor. Mediad, New York. 341.

15. Bartlett, G. R. 1959. Phosphorus assay in column chromatography. *J. Biol. Chem.* **234**: 466.

16. Matthews, C. M. E. 1957. The theory of tracer experiments with ^{131}I-labelled plasma proteins. *Phys. Med. Biol.* **2**: 36.

17. Nosslin, B. 1964. *In* Metabolism of Human Gamma Globulin (γ_{ss}-globulin). S. B. Anderson, editor. Scientific Publications, Ltd., Oxford.

18. Berson, S. A., and R. S. Yalow. 1957. Distribution and metabolism of I[131]-labeled proteins in man. *Fed. Proc.* **16**: 13s.

19. Volwiler, W., P. D. Goldsworthy, M. P. MacMartin, P. A. Wood, I. R. MacKay, and G. Fremont-Smith. 1955. Biosynthetic determination with radioactive sulfur of turn-over rates of various plasma proteins in normal and cirrhotic man. *J. Clin. Invest.* **34**: 1126.

20. Gitlin, D., D. G. Cornwell, D. Nikasato, J. L. Oncley, W. L. Hughes, Jr., and C. A. Janeway. 1958. Studies on metabolism of plasma proteins in nephrotic syndrome. II. Lipoproteins. *J. Clin. Invest.* **37**: 172.

21. Walton, V. W., P. J. Scott, J. Verrier Jones, R. F.

Fletcher, and T. Whitehead. 1963. Studies on low density lipoprotein turnover in relation to atromid therapy. *J. Atheroscler. Res.* **3**: 396.

22. Walton, K. W., P. J. Scott, P. W. Dykes, and J. W. L. Davies. 1965. Alterations of metabolism and turnover of I^{131} low density lipoprotein in myxoedema and thyrotoxicosis. *Clin. Sci. (London).* **29**: 217.

23. Scott, P. J., and C. C. Winterbourn. 1967. Low-density lipoprotein accumulation in actively growing xanthomas. *J. Atheroscler. Res.* **7**: 267.

24. Hurley, P. J., and P. J. Scott. 1970. Plasma turnover of S_f 0-9 low-density lipoprotein in normal men and women. *J. Atheroscler. Res.* **11**: 51.

25. McFarlane, A. S., D. Todd, and S. Cromwell. 1964. Fibrinogen catabolism in humans. *Clin. Sci. (London).* **26**: 415.

26. Barth, W. F., R. D. Wochner, T. A. Waldmann, and J. L. Fahey. 1964. Metabolism of human gamma macroglobulins. *J. Clin. Invest.* **43**: 1036.

27. Langer, T., R. I. Levy, and D. S. Fredrickson. 1969. Dietary and pharmacologic perturbation of beta lipoprotein (βLP) turnover. *Circulation.* **40**:(Suppl. III) 14.

28. Waldmann, T. A., and W. Strober. 1969. Metabolism of immunoglobulins. *Prog. Allergy.* **13**: 1.

29. Scott, P. J., and P. J. Hurley. 1969. Effect of clofibrate on low-density lipoprotein turnover in essential hypercholesterolaemia. *J. Atheroscler. Res.* **9**: 25.

30. Freeman, T. 1965. Gamma globulin metabolism in normal humans and in patients. *Ser. Haematol.* **4**: 76.

31. Langer, T., and R. I. Levy. 1970. Effect of nicotinic acid on beta lipoprotein metabolism. *Clin. Res.* **18**: 458.

32. Levy, R. I., T. Langer, A. M. Gotto, and D. S. Fredrickson. 1970. Familial hypobetalipoproteinemia: a defect in lipoprotein synthesis. *Clin. Res.* **18**: 539.

33. Lees, R. S., and E. H. Ahrens, Jr. 1969. Fat transport in abetalipoproteinemia: the effects of repeated infusions of beta-lipoprotein-rich plasma. *N. Engl. J. Med.* **280**: 1261.

34. Hellman, L., R. S. Rosenfeld, M. L. Eidinoff, D. K. Fukushima. T. F. Gallagher, C-I. Wang, and D. Adlersberg. 1955. Isotopic studies of plasma cholesterol of endogenous and exogenous origins. *J. Clin. Invest.* **34**: 48.

35. Gee, D. J., J. Goldstein, C. H. Gray, and J. F. Fowler. 1959. Biosynthesis of cholesterol in familial hypercholesterolaemic xanthomatosis. *Brit. Med. J.* **2**: 341.

36. Lewis, B., and N. B. Myant. 1967. Studies in the metabolism of cholesterol in subjects with normal plasma cholesterol levels and in patients with essential hypercholesterolaemia. *Clin. Sci. (London).* **32**: 201.

37. Goodman, D. S., and R. P. Noble. 1968. Turnover of plasma cholesterol in man. *J. Clin. Invest.* **47**: 231.

38. Grundy, S. M., and E. H. Ahrens, Jr. 1969. Measurements of cholesterol turnover, synthesis and absorption in man carried out by isotope kinetic and sterol balance methods. *J. Lipid Res.* **10**: 91.

39. Nestel, P. J., P. M. Whyte, and D. S. Goodman. 1969. Distribution and turnover of cholesterol in humans. *J. Clin. Invest.* **48**: 982.

Mutation and Cancer:
Statistical Study of Retinoblastoma

ALFRED G. KNUDSON, JR.

The origin of cancer by a process that involves more than one discreet stage is supported by experimental, clinical, and epidemiological observations. These stages are, in turn, attributed by many investigators to somatic mutations. Ashley (1) has calculated that the common cancers are produced by a number of mutations that varies from 3–7, according to the specific cancer. It was pointed out by Ashley that cancer could still be a process occurring in two physiologically different stages, as suggested by studies in chemical carcinogenesis, the number of mutations involved in each stage varying from cancer to cancer. What is lacking, however, is direct evidence that cancer can ever arise in as few as two steps and that each step can occur at a rate that is compatible with accepted values for mutation rates. Data are presented herein in support of the hypothesis that at least one cancer (the retinoblastoma observed in children) is caused by two mutational events.

PATIENT DATA

The records of all retinoblastoma patients admitted to the M. D. Anderson Hospital, some 48 cases during the period 1944–1969, were reviewed. These cases are tabulated (Table 1) with respect to unilaterality or bilaterality, sex, age at diagnosis, and family history. Whenever possible, the number of tumors in each eye was estimated.

DISCUSSION

Several authors have concluded that retinoblastoma may be caused by either a germinal or a somatic mutation (2–5). The fraction of cases inheriting the mutation may be estimated indirectly. The percentage of all cases that are bilateral is approximately 25–30 (5), the present series being higher (48%) than that because of referral bias. All bilateral cases should be counted as hereditary because the proportion of affected offspring closely approximates the 50% expected with dominant inheritance (5). On the other hand, of the 70–75% of all cases that are unilateral, only 15–20% are thought to be hereditary (3, 5); thus, 10–15% of all cases are unilateral and hereditary. The percentage of all retinoblastoma patients with the hereditary form is, therefore, in the range 35–45; among these, 25–40% are unilateral and 60–75% are bilateral. In contrast, 55–65% of all retinoblastoma cases are of the nonhereditary form and all are unilateral. These distributions are summarized in Table 2.

Some patients that inherit the gene for retinoblastoma are never affected, although they transmit the trait to offspring who may become affected. The size of this group is difficult to estimate. Previous estimates range generally from 1–20%. Some authors have probably overcorrected for ascertainment bias. The estimate by Falls and Neel (2) of a range 1.5–10% represents an attempt to avoid this bias.

If the above estimates are correct, then carriers of the germinal mutation are distributed as follows:

Unaffected	1–10%
Unilateral	25–40%
Bilateral	60–75%

These data strongly suggest the possibility that tumors are distributed in accord with a Poisson distribution. If the Poisson distribution is followed, the mean number of tumors, m, formed per gene carrier may be estimated.

The necessary calculation is complicated by the fact that more than one tumor can occur per eye and that multiple tumors may appear unilaterally. For mean numbers of tumors of one–five, the fractions that should by chance be unilateral and bilateral may be calculated as shown in Table 3. It is seen that $m = 3$ is the value most compatible with the distributions noted above for unaffected, unilaterally affected, and bilaterally affected carriers of the mutant gene.

This distribution of tumors additionally predicts a multiplicity distribution within affected hereditary cases. It is difficult to test this prediction because so many tumors are very large when seen and, in fact, this situation was true for

162

TABLE 1. Cases of retinoblastoma

(a) Bilateral cases

Case	Hospital number	Sex	Age at diagnosis (months)	No. of tumors right	No. of tumors left	Family history
1	03712	F	8	*	*	no
2	11571	M	3	*	*	no
3	12163	F	11	*	*	no
4	17076	M	2	*	1	no
5	18025	M	60	1	*	affected sib.
6	18237	M	22	*	*	no
7	20291	F	4	3	*	no
8	22699	F	18	2	*	no
9	24729	F	30	*	*	no
10	30464	M	3	2	1	no
11	30470	F	6	*	2	no
12	37837	M	7	*	*	affected sib.
13	41134	M	9	3	*	no
14	43391	F	4	5	*	no
15	44176	F	13	*	*	no
16	44649	M	18	*	4	no
17	46860	F	24	*	*	no
18	59704	F	44	1	*	no
19	67024	F	5	*	*	no
20	68422	M	12	*	1	no
21	69224	M	3	*	*	no
22	72656	M	12	*	1	no
23	74616	M	15	1	*	father and paternal uncle

(b) Unilateral cases

Case	Hospital number	Sex	Age at diagnosis (months)	No. of tumors	Family history
24	00198	F	48	*	no
25	03705	M	22	*	no
26	06600	M	33	*	no
27	08847	M	38	*	no
28	08997	F	47	*	no
29	19118	M	50	*	no
30	24986	M	32	*	no
31	26961	M	28	*	no
32	33131	F	31	*	no
33	36322	F	29	*	no
34	40061	F	21	*	no
35	40306	M	46	*	no
36	41628	F	36	*	no
37	45583	F	73	*	no
38	46371	M	29	*	no
39	47070	F	15	*	no
40	52892	M	52	*	no
41	54321	M	24	*	no
42	61533	M	8	*	no
43	64465	F	19	*	no
44	64622	M	36	*	no
45	68543	F	34	*	no
46	69502	F	27	*	no
47	74498	M	10	*	no
48	76092	F	8	*	no

* Number of tumors not determined.

163

all of our unilateral cases, for both eyes in nine of the bilateral cases, and for one eye in the remaining bilateral cases. However, a tumor count was possible in one eye of each of 14 bilateral cases (Table 1). The expected numbers for one eye among bilateral cases may be calculated from the binomial distribution, when terms of the unilateral (o,r and r,o) classes are eliminated, and are shown in Table 4. In the last columns of Table 4 are shown the numbers of tumors observed in single eyes in our 14 cases and in 52 cases of retinoblastoma reported by Stallard (6). The data clearly fall between $m = 2$ and $m = 3$.

This calculation permits another; namely, that of the probability that a mutant cell will develop into a tumor. If n is the total number of cells in the two retinae that have the potential for tumor formation, then m/n expresses the probability that a cell with the inherited mutation will develop into a tumor cell. The retinoblastoma is derived from a cell that generates both the inner neuroblastic layer (which gives rise to the ganglion and amacrine cells) and the outer neuroblastic layer (which gives rise to the bipolar, horizontal, and visual receptor cells). The order of magnitude of the number of retinoblasts is probably reflected by the order of magnitude of the number of ganglion cells, cells derived from the early-differentiated inner molecular layer. The number of ganglion cells has been estimated at 2×10^6 per retina, or 4×10^6 for two eyes (7). Using this value as an approximation for n, we find that the probability (m/n) that a cell with the inherited mutation will develop into a tumor cell is 0.75×10^{-6}. Since a majority of hereditary cases occurs within the first 2 years

TABLE 2. *Distribution of retinoblastoma cases by type and laterality (3, 5)*

	Bilateral	Unilateral	Total
Hereditary	25–30%	10–15%	35–45%
Nonhereditary	0	55–65%	55–65%
Total	25–30%	70–75%	100%

of prenatal and postnatal life, the probability, expressed as a mutation rate per year at either member of an autosomal gene pair, would be one-fourth of this value, or approximately 2×10^{-7} per year. This estimates the rate of a second mutation in cells already abnormal as a result of an inherited mutation at another gene site.

164

TABLE 3. *Expected distributions of tumors for various mean numbers*

Total tumors both eyes (r)	Probability (Poisson)	Fraction unilateral $2(1/2)^r$	Frequencies for various values of m				
			1	2	3	4	5
0	e^{-m}	···	0.368	0.135	0.050	0.018	0.007
1	me^{-m}	1	0.368/0*	0.271/0	0.150/0	0.073/0	0.034/0
2	$\dfrac{m^2e^{-m}}{2!}$	$1/2$	0.092/0.092	0.135/0.135	0.112/0.112	0.073/0.073	0.042/0.042
3	$\dfrac{m^3e^{-m}}{3!}$	$1/4$	0.015/0.046	0.045/0.135	0.056/0.168	0.049/0.147	0.034/0.131
4	$\dfrac{m^4e^{-m}}{4!}$	$1/8$	0.002/0.013	0.011/0.079	0.021/0.147	0.024/0.172	0.021/0.148
5	$\dfrac{m^5e^{-m}}{5!}$	$1/16$	0.000/0.003	0.002/0.034	0.006/0.095	0.010/0.147	0.011/0.158
6	$\dfrac{m^6e^{-m}}{6!}$	$1/32$	0.000/0.001	0.000/0.012	0.002/0.049	0.003/0.101	0.004/0.136
7	$\dfrac{m^7e^{-m}}{7!}$	$1/64$	···	0.000/0.003	0.000/0.022	0.001/0.059	0.002/0.098
$\geqq 8$	$\displaystyle\sum_{r=8}^{r=\infty}\dfrac{m^re^{-m}}{r!}$	$2(1/2)^r$	···	0.000/0.001	0.000/0.010	0.000/0.050	0.000/0.132
Totals: none			0.368	0.135	0.050	0.018	0.007
unilateral			0.477	0.464	0.347	0.233	0.148
bilateral			0.155	0.399	0.603	0.749	0.845

* Unilateral/bilateral.

Unilateral cases that do not result from germinal mutations constitute 55–65% of the total cases. If these cases arise by mutations at the same sites as in the hereditary form, then what is the relation between the somatic and germinal mutation rates for the first mutation? Let the two rates for this first mutation be μ_g (germinal) and μ_s (somatic), and the probability of the second event be m/n for both cases. Furthermore, let i be the total incidence of retinoblastoma, f_h the fraction of the hereditary cases, f_n the fraction of nonhereditary cases, q the population frequency of the germinal mutant gene, and s the coefficient of selection for the germinal mutant gene. Then the incidence of hereditary cases is:

$$f_h \cdot i = 2q(1 - e^{-m}).$$

Since $\mu_g = sq$, then

$$f_h \cdot i = 2\mu_g(1 - e^{-m})/s,$$

and

$$\mu_g = s \cdot f_h \cdot i/2(1 - e^{-m}).$$

The incidence of nonhereditary cases, $f_n \cdot i$, is equal to the product of the probability of the first mutation in somatic cells in the first year of fetal and postnatal life, $2\mu_s \cdot n$, and the probability of the second event, m/n, from which

$$f_n \cdot i = 2\mu_s \cdot n \cdot m/n = 2\mu_s \cdot m,$$

and

$$\mu_s = f_n \cdot i/2m.$$

The relationship between mutation rates is therefore:

$$\mu_s/\mu_g = f_n/f_h \cdot 1/ms \cdot (1 - e^{-m}).$$

An estimate of s is difficult, as it has become lower with therapeutic success. For purposes of this calculation, we assume a value of $s = 0.5$. Using this and values noted above for the other parameters, we calculate

$$\frac{\mu_s}{\mu_g} = \frac{0.60}{0.40} \cdot \frac{1}{(3)(0.5)} \cdot (0.95) \approx 1.$$

It is apparent that the two mutation rates are of a similar order of magnitude.

The incidence of retinoblastoma is approximately 5×10^{-5}, from which the germinal mutation rate, μ_g, may be calculated:

$$\mu_g = \frac{f_h \cdot i \cdot s}{2(1 - e^{-m})} = \frac{(0.4)(5 \times 10^{-5})(0.5)}{(2)(0.95)} =$$

$$5 \times 10^{-6} \text{ per generation.}$$

Tumors, one eye	Expected frequencies (%)				Observed		Observed frequency
					numbers		frequency
	$m = 1$	$m = 2$	$m = 3$	$m = 4$	14 cases, present series	52 cases, Stallard (6)	66 cases (%)
1	77	59	43	32	7	28	53
2	20	29	33	31	3	14	26
3	3	10	17	21	2	7	14
4		2.5	6	11	1	3	6
5			1.8	4.2	1		1.5

* The frequencies of bilateral tumors for various values of r and m are obtained from Table 3. The relative distribution of tumors between right (d) and left (s) eyes is obtained from the binomial expansion, $(d/2 + s/2)^r$. On multiplication, one obtains the expected distribution of tumors among bilateral cases, as illustrated for $m = 1$:

r	Frequency, bilateral (Table 2)	Frequency of tumors one eye			
		1	2	3	4
2	0.092	0.092			
3	0.046	0.023	0.023		
4	0.013	0.004	0.006	0.004	
5	0.003	0.000	0.001	0.001	0.000
	Totals	0.119	0.030	0.005	
	Per cent	77	20	3	

This rate is close to that of $6–7 \times 10^{-6}$ calculated by Vogel (3). In the nonhereditary form, the mutation rate is expressed per year, which, assuming a generation time of 25–30 years, yields an estimate of approximately 2×10^{-7} per year.

Although the above data are incompatible with two *independent* mutational "second events", they do not constitute direct evidence that a single independent "event" of any kind is involved. If a second, single event is involved, the distribution of bilateral cases with time should be an exponential function, i.e., the fraction of the total cases that develops in a given period of time should be constant, as expressed in the relationship $dS/dt = -kS$, and $\ln S = -kt$, where S is the fraction of survivors not yet diagnosed at time t, and dS is the change in this fraction in the interval dt. As shown in Fig. 1, this is indeed the case. By contrast, the fractional decrease in unilateral cases per unit time does not show this relationship (Fig. 1). Although 15–20% of the unilateral cases should be of the hereditary type and so contaminate the data, the observations more nearly fit the anticipated two-mutation expression, ln $S = -kt^2$, derived by Burch (8). That a difference in mean age at diagnosis exists between unilateral and bilateral cases has been noted previously. The respective mean ages at diagnosis for bilateral and unilateral cases have been reported in other series as 15 and 24 months (9) and 15 and 29 months (10), and in the present series are 15 and 32 months.

The exponential decline in new hereditary cases with time reflects the occurrence of a second event at a constant rate in a declining population of embryonal cells. For the nonhereditary cases, this declining population of cells must experience two independently occurring events. New cases of both types occur only in childhood because the embryonal cells vanish.

The data presented here and in the literature are consistent with the hypothesis that at least one cancer, retinoblastoma, can be caused by two mutations, each of which occurs at a rate of the order of 2×10^{-7} per year. One of these mutations may be inherited as a result of a previous germinal mutation that occurs at about the same rate. Those patients that inherit one mutation develop tumors earlier than do those who develop the nonhereditary form of the disease; in a majority of cases those who inherit a mutation develop more than one tumor. On the other hand, the probability that an individual not inheriting a mutation would develop more than one tumor is vanishingly small, so that nonhereditary cases are invariably unifocal.

The two-mutation hypothesis is consistent with current thought on the mutational origin of cancer. Ashley (1) has reviewed two-hit and multiple-hit theories of carcinogenesis and concluded that the common cancers are produced by about 3–7 mutations. Interestingly, one of the lowest estimates was for brain tumors, which are, like retinoblastoma, derived from neural elements. Ashley suggests that the two-stage hypothesis of initiation and promotion may still be correct, in that each stage may result from more than one mutation.

In the present series of 48 cases, three, all bilateral, are familial. In one case an affected father and his affected brother had unaffected parents. The same situation of affected sibs with unaffected parents exists for our other two cases. Such instances have been noted repeatedly in the past, the most dramatic report being that of Macklin (11), who found not only four families resembling those in the present series, but

168

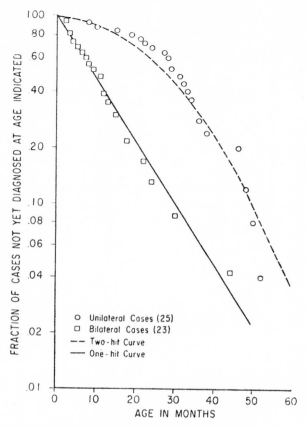

FIG. 1. Semilogarithmic plot of fraction of cases of retinoblastoma not yet diagnosed (S) vs. age in months (t). The one-hit curve was calculated from $\log S = -t/30$, the two-hit curve from $\log S = -4 \times 10^{-4} t^2$.

also ten families with affected cases in more widely separated relationships. Occasionally an unaffected parent may actually have had a retinoblastoma that has undergone spontaneous regression, but this must happen very rarely (2). On the other hand, if one attempts to attribute these occurrences to decreased penetrance, an inconsistency develops. Prior to the appearance of cases in a branch of a family, penetrance is very low; after its occurrence, penetrance is very high. As pointed out by Neel (12), this circumstance is precisely that discussed by Auerbach (13) with respect to the dominantly inherited split hand, or lobster claw, deformity. Auerbach compared this pattern with that found in *Drosophila*, in response to chemical mutagenesis by nitrogen mustard, and refers to it as an example of delayed mutation, or premutation.

1. Ashley, D. J. B., *Brit. J. Cancer*, **23,** 313 (1969).
2. Falls, H. F., and J. V. Neel, *Arch. Ophthalmol.*, **46,** 367 (1951).
3. Vogel, F., *Z. Menschl. Vererb. Konstit-Lehre*, **34,** 205 (1957).
4. Smith, S. M., and A. Sorsby, *Ann. Hum. Genet.*, **23,** 50 (1958).
5. Schappert-Kimmijser, J., G. D. Hemmes, and R. Nijland, *Ophthalmologica*, **151,** 197 (1966).
6. Stallard, H. B., *Tr. Ophth. Soc. U.K.*, **82,** 473 (1962).
7. Van Buren, J. M., in *The Retinal Ganglion Cell Layer* (Charles C Thomas, Springfield, Ill., 1963), p. 64.
8. Burch, P. R. J., *Proc. Roy. Soc.*, **162 B,** 223 (1965).
9. Leelawongs, N., and C. D. J. Regan, *Amer. J. Ophthalmol.*, **66,** 1050 (1968).
10. Jensen, O. A., *Acta Ophthalmol.*, **43,** 821 (1965).
11. Macklin, M. T., *Amer. J. Hum. Genet.*, **12,** 1 (1960).
12. Neel, J. V., in *Methodology in Human Genetics*, ed. W. J. Burdette (Holden-Day, San Francisco, 1962), p. 203.
13. Auerbach, C., *Ann. Hum. Genet.*, **20,** 266 (1956).

Quantitative Abnormalities of Allotypic Genes
in Families with Primary Immune Deficiencies

STEPHEN D. LITWIN AND H. HUGH FUDENBERG

Members of the families of individuals with adult onset of primary hypogammaglobulinemia often have abnormalities in the amount of serum immunoglobulin and in the response of peripheral blood lymphocytes to mitogenic stimulation, as well as frequent clinical problems (1, 2). These observations suggest that this immunologic disorder involves a genetic defect; however, analyses have failed to reveal a clear mode of inheritance. Recent reports have noted a failure of allelic expression in family members. Quantitative measurements of the immunoglobulin antigens were not available,

---

Abbreviations: IgG, immunoglobulin G; IgG1, immunoglobulin G1; IgG2, immunoglobulin G2; IgG3, immunoglobulin G3; IgG4, immunoglobulin G4; Gm factors, genetic antigens of human immunoglobulin G; SD, standard deviation.

‡ Human sera contain four IgG subclasses (IgG1, IgG2, IgG3, IgG4). Gm(a) and Gm(f) are Gm genetic factors for antithetical structural genes for IgG1 heavy chains. Gm(g) and Gm(b) are similarly Gm markers for antithetical genes of IgG3 chains. The numerical designation for the Gm antigens is as follows: Gm(a) = (1); Gm(f) = (4); Gm(g) = 21; Gm(b) = (5); Gm(z) = (17).

but the possibility of a defective regulatory gene was nonetheless raised on the basis of altered phenotypic expression (3).

A recently developed method for quantitative measurement of human IgG allotypes (Gm factors)‡ permits detailed analysis of Gm gene products (4, 5). This method is particularly useful for the study of individuals who are heterozygous at the IgG gene loci, for which test reagents that detect antithetical Gm markers are available (6). The selected families included three principal pedigrees (SP, STR, and DE) containing heterozygotes for IgG1 and IgG3 heavy chains in three generations.

The primary purpose of the study was to determine whether members of the families of certain patients with primary immunodeficiency had quantitative allotype aberrations suggesting they were carriers of defective genes. The frequent appearance in certain families of disproportionate amounts of Gm antigens permitted analysis of the pattern of segregation of allotype defects; evaluation of these data suggested certain postulates (see *Discussion*) regarding the nature of the genetic abnormality.

MATERIALS AND METHODS

67 Sera from selected families were tested (age and sex of subjects, all Caucasians, are listed in Table 1). All probands were adults diagnosed as having primary variable immunodeficiency, with the exception of family RE (7). The RE proband was a 6-year-old boy, who, because of his relatively high IgG and the lack of immune deficiency in other male relatives, was not a typical case of X-linked hypogammaglobulinemia. One other member of family STR (II$_2$, see Fig. 2) also had primary hypogammaglobulinemia. None of the subjects had received recent blood transfusions or γ-globulin therapy. Routine Gm typing in test tubes was performed on all samples for Gm(a), (b^0), (f), (z), and (g), as described (8). To be sure that low amounts of Gm antigen were not overlooked, all homozygous samples were tested undiluted as well as at the usual 1:10 dilution. IgG, IgM, IgA, and kappa and lambda light chains were measured by the radial diffusion method with monospecific antiserum (9, 10). Cellulose acetate electrophoresis and immunoelectrophoresis were performed by routine methods.

After initial Gm typing, quantitation of the concentrations of the various Gm allotypes was performed in duplicate by a modified hemagglutination inhibition assay with an Autoanalyzer (Technicon, Tarrytown, N.Y.). Standards for Gm antigens were isolated IgG myeloma proteins of the appropriate genetic types. Protein concentrations were measured by the Folin method; standards were carefully tested for purity by microimmunoelectrophoresis and double-diffusion in agar, as well as by the more sensitive hemagglutination titration for contaminating Gm antigens associated with normal IgG. Previous studies with this assay have established that quantitative results do not vary with Gm agglutinators of similar specificity. The reagents used and the technical details of the method have been described (4, 5, 11). The lower limit for detection of Gm was 0.09 mg/ml. A Caucasian population of 157 sera, obtained from the New York Blood Center (courtesy of Dr. F. H. Allen, Jr.), was used to determine the mean concentration and range for each phenotype population. The ±1 SD for the Gm(f)/Gm(a) ratio was obtained from the heterozygotes of this group. Allelic imbalance was defined as present when the Gm(f)/Gm(a) ratio of a heterozygous serum was less than 0.44 or greater than 1.92 (i.e., ±2 SD from the 1.17 mean of the normal population) (11). Serum values for each phenotype are listed in Table 1. Results obtained for allelic concentrations are consistent with published data on IgG subclass antigens in Caucasian sera (12–14).

RESULTS

Seven sera from the SP, STR, and DE families out of 27 heterozygous samples tested had an imbalance in the concentrations of allelic IgG1 gene products (these sera are *italicized* in Table 1). Three of these sera (SP I_1, SP III_1, and STR III_1) had amounts of one Gm factor 2 SD below the phenotype mean and were absolutely deficient. The remaining four abnormal samples had allelic imbalance, as reflected in the distorted Gm(f)/Gm(a) ratio. This latter finding indicated a disparity between the expressions of isoallelic IgG1 genes, that was much greater than that characteristic of the normal control population of heterozygotes (Table 1) (11).

The possibility that a monoclonal population of immunoglobulin molecules was responsible for the discrepancy in allelic concentrations was considered. The seven samples were examined by cellulose acetate electrophoresis and immunoelectrophoresis against specific IgG1, IgG3, IgG4, Fd, Fab, κ (kappa-type immunoglobulin light chains), and λ (λ-type immunoglobulin light chains) antisera. There was no restricted electrophoretic or immunoelectrophoretic distribution. Kappa/lambda ratios of three samples (family SP I_1, III_1 and family STR III_1) were normal. The concentrations of the IgG1 and IgG3 subclasses were determined in these sera and were consistent with the Gm values.

A second explanation of the discordant concentrations of allelic gene products is a quantitative variability in the ex-

173

TABLE 1. *Sera Gm and immunoglobulin concentrations of families of subjects with primary immune deficiency*

Test samples*	Gm allotypes (mg/ml)				Ratio Gm(f)/Gm(a)	Immunoglobulin classes¶ (mg/ml)		
	Gm(f)	Gm(a)	Gm(b)	Gm(g)		IgG	IgA	IgM
					$1.17 \pm$	$1158 \pm$	$200 \pm$	$99 \pm$
	3.52 ± 1.14	2.99 ± 0.95	0.86 ± 0.50	0.28 ± 0.12	0.37‡	305	61	27
					$(0.43-$	$(569-$	$(61-$	$(47-$
					$1.91)$	$1919)$	$330)$	$147)$
Phenotype†								
Gm(f+a+b+g+)	3.52 ± 1.14	2.99 ± 0.95	0.86 ± 0.50	0.28 ± 0.12				
Gm(f+a−b+g−)	6.70 ± 1.56	0	1.25 ± 0.65	0				
Gm(f−a+b−g+)	0	5.28 ± 1.22	0	0.52 ± 0.24				
SP family								
I₁ M	8.70	0.40	0.23	<0.1	20+	14.0	0.68	1.36
I₂ F	3.70	0	1.07	0		9.7	2.02	0.99
II₁ Prob (35M)	0.64	0.26	0.21	<0.1	2.46	3.4	0	0
II₂ Sp	4.40	2.80	1.45	0.45	1.57	14.2	0.86	2.30
II₃ B	7.50	0	0.94	0		16.7	1.60	2.65
III₁ S (10)	0.30	2.80	0.24	0.47	0.10	5.4	0.98	0.79
III₂ D (9)	6.00	0	0.87	0		7.6	0.68	1.30
III₃ S (8)	8.00	0	1.07	0		10.5	0.51	0.57
III₄ S (7)	3.32	2.00	0.34	0.10	1.66	6.9	0.68	0.90
III₅ D (5)	3.62	1.64	0.46	0.27	2.21	9.1	0.74	0.79
STR family								
I₁ M	8.40	2.80	0.98	0.29	2.21	12.9	1.97	0.78
II₁ Prob (45M)	0.19	0.12	NT	0		0.66	0	0
II₂ B	<0.1	<0.1	<0.1	<0.1				
II₃ B	10.4	0	0.81	0		11.9	2.01	1.28
II₄ Sil	5.2	0	0.81	0		9.7	0.81	0.41
III₁ D (12)	11.2	1.02	0.26	0.22	9.33	14.2	2.42	0.87

III_4	Niece	8.8	0	0.56	0		10.4	0.81	0.73
III_5	Niece	6.0	0	0.66	0		7.1	0.88	0.82
DE family									
I_1	M (77)	9.1	2.7	0.51	0.22	*3.37*	14.3	0.40	0.70
II_1	Sis (45)	10.1	0	1.62	0		13.8	0.91	0.81
II_2	Sis (48)	5.70	4.25	0.78	<0.1	1.34	12.0	1.05	1.30
II_3	Prob (33M)	0.25	0.44	0.12	<0.1	0.57	0.75	0	0.15
II_4	Sp (32)	8.00	0	1.85	0		12.0	1.72	0.90
II_5	B (51)	5.26	2.32	0.62	0.23	*2.27*	14.7	1.90	1.10
II_6	B (38)	5.40	5.60	1.00	0.49	0.96	13.3	1.05	1.10
II_7	B (50)	10.50	0	0.96	0		14.0	0.18	1.30
III_1	D (7)	6.10	3.21	0.41	0.18	1.90	10.0	0.48	0.56
III_2	D (10)	11.20	0	1.20	0		13.5	0.84	0.76
RU family									
I_1	Aunt (73)	3.10	0	1.25	0	1.16	5.20	0.70	0.90
I_2	Aunt (70)	3.35	2.88	0.34	0.15		NT	NT	NT
I_3	Unc (76)	3.83	0	0.74	0		6.00	0.84	0.43
I_4	F (74)	3.35	0	1.05	0	0.95	5.20	1.25	0.46
I_5	M (73)	4.20	4.40	1.05	0.43	1.11	12.00	0	0.54
I_6	Unc (75)	3.35	3.00	1.15	0.32	0.87	4.10	2.75	0.25
II_1	Sp (45)	1.64	1.88	0.53	0.15	0.87	9.00	1.25	1.25
II_2	Prob (41M)	0.42	0	0.13	0.15		1.25	0	0.18
II_3	B (42)	1.40	1.68	0.47	0.15	0.83	4.00	0.42	0.34
III_1	D (20)	2.40	3.40	0.68	0.44	0.70	8.80	0	1.60
III_2	S (15)	2.72	2.52	0.40	0.16	1.08	7.20	0.36	1.75
III_3	D (17)	2.62	1.80	0.61	0.26	1.45	5.20	0	1.15
III_4	S (13)	2.72	0	0.60	0		5.50	0.70	0.88
DELA family									
I_1	M (45)	6.50	0	1.10	0		10.5	3.10	1.36
I_2	F (50)	12.60	0	1.22	0		18.6	NT	NT
II_1	Prob (21M)	0.48	0.74	0.1	<0.1	0.65	4.00	0.16	0.02
II_2	Sis (24)	14.2	0	2.45	0		18.50	3.10	3.00

TABLE 1. (Continued)

Test samples*	Gm allotypes (mg/ml)				Ratio Gm(f)/Gm(a) 1.17 ± 0.37‡ (0.43–1.91)	Immunoglobulin classes ¶ (mg/ml)		
	Gm(f)	Gm(a)	Gm(b)	Gm(g)		IgG 1158 ± 305 (569–1919)	IgA 200 ± 61 (61–300)	IgM 99 ± 27 (47–147)
JA family								
I₁ Prob (54F)	0.22	0.17	0.10	<0.1	1.3	1.0	0.19	0
I₂ Sp	4.04	0	0.98	0		8.9	2.05	0.46
II₁ D (25)	8.00	0	0.79	0		15.5	1.50	1.50
II₂ D (28)	6.20	0	0.97	0		14.9	2.30	1.50
FR family								
I₁ F (67)	2.76	2.04	0.48	0.3	1.24	10.0	1.4	1.6
II₁ Prob (28M)	0.72	0.62	0.05	NT	1.35	1.5	0.13	0.18
II₂ Sp	4.95	0	0.90	0		6.9	NT	NT
III₁ S (15)	3.55	0	0.29	0		4.7	0.10	0.77
III₂ D (10)	3.12	2.08	0.30	<0.1	1.50	7.0	0.28	0.17
RT family								
I₁ Prob (53F)	0	0.28	0	<0.1		0.40	0.16	0.18
I₂ Sp	4.88	6.44	0.64	0.30	0.75	18.0	5.0	0.56
II₁ D	0	9.20	0	0.43		16.0	0	0.56
II₂ D	6.40	3.62	3.5	1.2	0.69	21.0	0	0.56
RE family								
I₁ M	2.88	2.38	0.97	0.30	1.21	10.7	2.25	0.76
II₁ Prob (6M)	0.78	0.65	<0.1	<0.1	1.20	2.1	0.70	0.22
II₂ B	5.55	0	NT	0		7.2		0.64
JO family								
I₁ M	0	5.20	0	0.42		11.50	1.35	0.99
II₁ Prob	0.24	0.90	<0.1	0.57	0.26	1.77	0	0.37
II₂ Sp	5.2	0	0.61	0		11.70	1.95	0.90
II₃ Sis	0	3.60	0	NT	NT	NT	NT	NT

* The following abbreviations were used for the family members: M = mother, F = father, Prob = proband with primary immune deficiency, B = brother, Sis = sister, S = son, D = daughter, Sp = spouse, Unc = uncle, Sil = sister-in-law.

† The three major phenotypes found in a normal Caucasian population (157 sera) and the mean ±SD sera concentrations are shown. Gm(f+a+b+g+) sera are heterozygous for Gmza,g/b,f; Gm(f+a−b+g−) and Gm(f−a−b−g+) sera are homozygous for Gmb,f/b,f and Gmg,za/g, za, respectively.

‡ The ratio of the mean ±SD sera concentrations of a normal Caucasian population is seen with the 2-SD range in parentheses. In the data given for each serum sample *italicized values* indicate a ratio significantly outside of the normal range.

¶ Mean ± SD (range) are shown below the class (9).

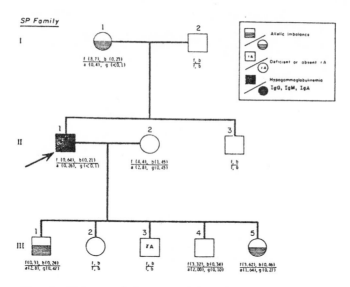

FIG. 1. Below each heterozygous subject, the Gm factors present and their sera concentrations in mg/ml are seen. An *arrow* indicates the proband.

pression of genes of the same allelic type, some being genetically "high" and others "low." The family data from this study do not support the genetic transmission of such genes (Figs. 1 and 2), nor do studies of normal families (11). *Thus, the most plausible explanation of the allelic imbalance is that one Gm gene is relatively or absolutely deficient.*

Three of the aberrant sera were from mothers of affected sons and raise the possibility of an X-linked defect. The maternal data are not attributable to random inactivation of genes on the X chromosome in females in accordance with the Lyon hypothesis, as control data from normal sera do not exhibit this finding (11). It should be noted, however, that two other affected families in this study have normal values for heterozygous maternal sera and, in family SP, the affected male propositus has a son with allotype abnormalities.

Detailed analysis of the SP and STR families provided information on the nature of the possible genetic defect (Figs. 1 and 2). Allelic imbalance appeared in three generations. In family SP, the serum of the mother of the affected man, I_1, had a very low concentration of Gm(a) and an excess of Gm(f); the paternal serum was homozygous for *Gmf* and had normal values. The small amount of IgG1 chains present in the proband's serum contained 2 to 3-fold more Gm(f+) than

177

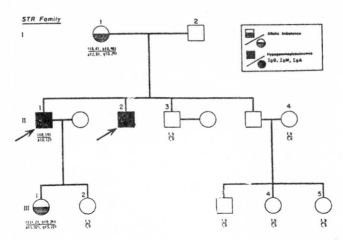

FIG. 2. Below each heterozygous subject, the Gm factors present and their sera concentrations in mg/ml are seen. An *arrow* indicates the proband.

Gm(a+) IgG. Of the proband's five children (III$_{1-5}$), two of three heterozygotes had allelic imbalance in opposite directions, while the remaining children had normal Gm measurements. The phenotypes in SP do not permit us to exclude the possibility that the father (I$_2$) contributed an abnormal *Gm*f gene, which in turn was transmitted to child III$_1$. Another explanation is that a regulatory (quantitative) defect is independent of the Gm structural genes. In contrast to family SP, in family STR both a parent and a child of the affected had depressed amounts of Gm(a) in their sera.

The presence of normal Gm values in many children and parents of probands is a general observation noted in this study. Seven of ten heterozygous children, three of four siblings, and three of six heterozygous parents, had normal Gm serum values (Table 1). Since most of these relatives would be obligatory carriers if the disorder were determined by two defective structural genes, these data are of critical importance, and weigh against a recessive mode of inheritance.

Not only were the gene products of antithetical genes (*Gm*a and *Gm*f) at the IgG1 locus examined, but also the concentrations of Gm(b) and Gm(g) at the IgG3 locus. In III$_1$ of family SP, Gm(b) was lower than Gm(g); this was the only serum in the study group in which this was found. This is of interest, since Gm(a) was elevated in this serum, and *Gm*a and *Gm*g are linked in Caucasians. The remaining samples have Gm(b) > Gm(g), as is characteristic of normal sera (11).

178

The RU family appears to constitute a special situation and probably reflects the heterogeneity within the present, admittedly unsatisfactory, clinical classification of "variable immunodeficiency." The low amounts of IgG, IgA, and IgM in many of the relatives suggest that they are carriers, but this could not be confirmed for IgG by study of the allotypes of informative heterozygotes. The striking lack of aberrations of Gm concentrations in this pedigree, in comparison to the other principal families, serves as a control in some respects.

Other immune aberrations previously described in association with primary hypogammaglobulinemia were noted in these families, in particular the deficiency of IgA.

DISCUSSION

Selective allotype abnormalities of IgG1 in close relatives of affected individuals are consistent with the suggestion that many cases of primary immunodeficiency of adult onset are hereditary. Previous data support this view. In 1962 Fudenberg et al. noted serum immunologic abnormalities in family studies of "acquired" agammaglobulinemia (1); other workers subsequently described similar families. Phytohemagglutinin-stimulated lymphocytes of affected subjects and their parents were shown to be abnormal with respect to DNA, RNA, and protein synthesis (2). Families with decreased or absent Gm factors and IgG subclasses have been described (3). Selective disturbances of immunoglobulin classes and IgG subclasses in patients and, in certain instances, also in family members (13), have been observed in some patients. Since each subclass and its alleles are presumably determined at a separate locus, the pattern of involvement is consistent with a disturbance at the genetic level. It can be argued that an alternative possibility is an infectious agent producing the reported familial clustering of abnormalities. The present Gm data do not support this view, since spouses of affected subjects had normal allotype concentrations (Table 1). Further, several of the relatives with allotype aberrations lived great distances from the probands for up to 20 years before the onset of the disease. Thus, the cumulative evidence indicates a genetic component in this disorder, and raises the question as to whether structural or regulatory genes are involved.

The possibility of a recessive structural gene abnormality was analyzed in heterozygous relatives; they would be obligatory carriers if such a theory were correct. Evaluation depends on the measurement of both the concentration of the products of the allelic genes and the determination of the balance between alleles. Since gene products of both allelic genes can be distinguished, even a single deficient gene should present unambiguous data in carriers. Although over a quarter of the relatives had abnormalities, this is lower than the 75% plus figure needed to fit a simple recessive structural gene hypothesis. Yount *et al.* (13), as well as other workers, have noted that in certain pedigrees an affected proband may transmit the capacity to synthesize qualitatively and quantatively normal IgG1 molecules. A final objection to the presence of abnormal structural genes is the large number of loci that determine the synthesis of immunoglobulins. It is difficult to explain how several structural loci could be affected.

In view of the difficulties inherent in any structural gene hypothesis, a regulatory gene abnormality must be considered. Supportive evidence includes the quantitative rather than qualitative nature of the abnormality noted in relatives in this present study, the limited rather than absent immunoglobulins found in all patients with hypogammaglobulinemia, the reports of reversible Gm genome suppression (3), and the selective involvement of IgG loci and allelic genes (13). Useful data are suggested in a recent report of partial aminoacid analysis of H(heavy) and L(light) immunoglobulin chains of five patients with adult onset of hypogammaglobulinemia (15). The postulated defect could involve regulator gene sites affecting "cis" loci or immunoglobulin gene "repressors" or "activators" that show allelic specificity. There is precedent for defects in regulatory mechanisms from the detailed work of Jacob and Monod on bacteria, but in mammals the action of such genes remains speculative (16). The present data extend current knowledge by emphasizing that *quantitative rather than qualitative abnormalities* predominate in these families. In view of the complexity of the regulation of immunoglobulin production, further data on antibody synthesis by the contiguous genes for IgG heavy chains is required.

The involvement of *Gm*a in one generation and *Gm*f in another generation of the SP family suggests that the presumed quantitative problem can *segregate independently of the Gm genes*. This unproven possibility would explain some of the present inconsistencies in current genetic interpretations.

It is clear that this poorly defined form of hypogammaglobulinemia includes several different clinical entities. The present data suggest that in some families the defect is a complex genetic problem involving control by regulatory genes.

The authors are grateful to Dr. Neil Goldberg for sera from the RU family. This research was supported in part by grants from the United States Public Health Service: AI-09239, AM-11796, AM-20122, AI-09145, and AM-08527.

This work was presented in part at the Meeting of the American Society of Clinical Investigation in Atlantic City, N.J., May, 1971.

1. Fudenberg, H. H., German, J. L., III & Kunkel, H. G. (1962) *Arthritis Rheum.* 5, 565–588.
2. Fudenberg, H. H., Kamin, R., Salmon, S. & Tormey, D. C. (1967) in *Nobel Symposium 3, "Gamma Globulins,"* ed. Killander, J. (Almqvist & Wiksell, Stockholm, Sweden), pp. 646–672.
3. Rivat, B. P. & Ropartz, C. (1969) *Humangenetik* 8, 183–194.
4. Litwin, S. D. (1969) *Vox Sang.* 17, 194.
5. Litwin, S. D. (1971) *J. Immunol.* 106, 589–597.
6. Natvig, J. B., Kunkel, H. G. & Litwin, S. D. (1967) *Cold Spring Harbor Symp. Quant. Biol.* 32, 173–180.
7. The terminology for primary immunodeficiencies is taken from W.H.O. report [Fudenberg, H. H., Good, R. A., Hitzig, W. H., *et al.* (1971) *Pediatrics* 47, 927 (1971)]. All patients in this study were classified as having primary variable immunodeficiency.
8. Grubb, R. (1970) in *The Genetic Markers of Human Immunoglobulins* (Springer-Verlag, New York and Heidelberg), pp. 5–8.
9. Stiehm, E. R. & Fudenberg, H. H. (1966) *Pediatrics* 37, 715–727.
10. Mancini, G., Carbonara, A. O. & Heremans, J. F. (1965) *Immunochemistry* 2, 235–254.
11. Litwin, S. D., & Balaban, S. (1972) *J. Immunol.* 108, 991–999.
12. Yount, W. J., Kunkel, H. G. & Litwin, S. D. (1967) *J. Exp. Med.* 125, 177–190.
13. Yount, W. J., Hong, R., Seligman, M., Good, R. & Kunkel, H. G. (1971) *J. Clin. Invest.* 49, 1957–1966.
14. Morell, A., Terry, W. D. & Waldmann, T. (1970) *J. Clin. Invest.* 49, 673–680.
15. Wang, A. C. & Fudenberg, H. H., *Meeting of Amer. Soc. of Hematology*, Dec., 1971.
16. Parker, W. C. & Bearn, A. G. (1963) *Amer. J. Med.* 34, 680–691.

Blood Enzymes in the de Lange Syndrome

G. F. SMITH, PARVIN JUSTICE, and D. Y. Y. HSIA

The de Lange syndrome is a clinical entity in which retardation of mental and physical development occurs in association with a number of other characteristic features, involving particularly the face and limbs (Berg et al, 1970). Dahlqvist, Hall, and Källén (1969) reported that galactose-1-phosphate uridyl transferase activity in red blood cells of patients with de Lange syndrome was elevated. More recently, Daniel and Higgins (1971) found increased serum α-ketoglutarate and serum glutamate levels in patients with the characteristic features of this syndrome. Since the aetiology and the pathophysiology of the de Lange syndrome has not been established it was decided that a careful look at the red and white blood cell enzymes was indicated in this syndrome.

Material and Methods

Ten to 20 ml of heparinized blood was obtained from patients and matched controls. The blood was sedimented in the cold for 45–90 minutes with 6% dextran in normal saline. These were mixed in a ratio of 1 ml of dextran per 5 ml of blood. The white cell rich supernatant was removed to within 0·2 cm of the red blood cells. For leucocyte glucose-6-phosphate dehydrogenase the blood was sedimented with 3% fibrinogen solution in Tris buffer pH 7·0 containing 50 mM β-mercaptoethanol.

Leucocyte and erythrocyte galactose-1-phosphate

It is with great regret that I have to report the death of Professor Hsia on 27 January 1972—Ed.

uridyl transferase were assayed according to the method of Mellman and Tedesco (1965).

The tests for glucose-6-phosphate dehydrogenase, acid phosphatase, and alkaline phosphatase were done with white cells prepared by washing with 0·2% saline to lyse the red cells. The white cells for acid phosphates and alkaline phosphates were lysed with 100 mg% solution of saponin in water. For the glucose-6-phosphate dehydrogenase, the white cells were lysed in Tris buffer 0·19 M pH 8 containing 10 mg% saponin and 0·4 mM TPN.

Erythrocyte glucose-6-phosphate dehydrogenase was assayed by the method of Zinkham (1959). Leucocyte glucose-6-phosphate dehydrogenase was assayed by the method of Shih et al (1965). Acid and alkaline phosphatase were assayed using p-nitrophenol phosphate as substrate (Bessey et al, 1946).

Results

The results of the enzyme studies are seen in Table I. While there were minor differences between the results of the de Lange and control groups, none is statistically significant.

In general, the values for the de Lange patients were more variable than those for the control group suggesting greater heterogeneity. However, there was no evidence of any consistent blood cell enzyme changes as has been described with certain other chromosomal disorders (Hsia et al, 1971).

This study was supported by a grant from the Mental Health Section of the State of Illinois and from the Association for the Aid of Crippled Children. We wish to thank Miss Nancy Becker for her technical assistance.

TABLE I

	Controls		De Lange	
	No.	Mean ± SD	No.	Mean ± SD
White blood cells				
Galactose-1-phosphate uridyl transferase (μM/hr/10⁶ WBC)	12	14·8 ± 3·1	11	18·5 ± 5·5
Glucose-6-phosphate dehydrogenase (μM/hr/10⁶ WBC)	5	1·08 ± 0·20	5	0·92 ± 0·22
Acid phosphatase (mg P/hr/mg protein)	11	147·0 ± 37·0	7	164·0 ± 35·0
Alkaline phosphatase (mg P/hr/mg protein)	11	8·4 ± 1·6	6	8·8 ± 3·5
Red blood cells				
Galactose-1-phosphate uridyl transferase (μM/hr/ml RBC)	12	5·7 ± 1·8	13	6·0 ± 2·0
Glucose-6-phosphate dehydrogenase (μM/hr/ml RBC)	8	1·69 ± 0·3	8	1·87 ± 0·49
6-Phosphogluconate dehydrogenase (μM/hr/ml RBC)	6	1·63 ± 0·31	6	1·92 ± 0·45

182

REFERENCES

Berg, J. M., McCreary, B. D., Ridler, M. A. C., and Smith, G. F. (1970). *The De Lange Syndrome*. Pergamon Press, Oxford.

Bessey, O. A., Lowry, O. H., and Brock, M. J. (1946). Method for rapid determination of alkaline phosphatase with 5 cubic milli-metres of serum. *Journal of Biological Chemistry*, **164**, 321–329.

Dahlqvist, A., Hall, B., and Källén (1969). Blood cell galactos-1-phosphate uridyl transferase activity in dysplastic patients, with and without chromosomal aberrations. *Human Heredity*, **19**, 628–640.

Daniel, W. L. and Higgins, J. V. (1971). Biochemical and genetic investigation of the De Lange syndrome. *American Journal of Diseases of Children*, **121**, 401–404.

Hsia, D. Y. Y., Justice, P., Smith, G. F., and Dowben, R. M. (1971) Down's syndrome. A critical review of the biochemical and immunological data. *American Journal of Diseases of Children*, **121**, 153–161.

Mellman, W. J. and Tedesco, T. A. (1965). An improved assay of erythrocyte and leukocyte galactose-1-phosphate uridyl trans-ferase: stabilization of the enzyme by a thiol protective reagent. *Journal of Laboratory and Clinical Medicine*, **66**, 980–986.

Shih, L. Y., Wong, P., Inouye, T., Makler, M., and Hsia, D. Y. Y. (1965). Enzymes in Down's syndrome. *Lancet*, **2**, 746–747.

Zinkham, W. H. (1959). An in-vitro abnormality of glutathione metabolism in erythrocytes from normal newborns: mechanism and clinical significance. *Pediatrics*, **23**, 18–32.

Low dopamine-ß-hydroxylase activity in Down's syndrome

L. WETTERBERG, K.-H. GUSTAVSON, M. BÄCKSTRÖM, S. B. ROSS AND Ö. FRÖDÉN

The low serotonin concentration in whole blood reported in patients with Down's syndrome and indicating a disturbance of the metabolism of biogenic amines (Rosner et al. 1965, Bazelon et al. 1967) prompted a study of a possible disturbance also in the catecholamine metabolism.

In this letter we report that patients with Down's syndrome have a decreased activity of plasma dopamine-β-hydroxylase (DBH), the enzyme that is responsible for forming noradrenaline from dopamine.

DBH was assayed in plasma following the method of Weinshilboum & Axelrod (1971 a). The plasma was stored at $-20°C$ until assayed. Under this condition no change in DBH activity was observed.

The results in Table 1 show that children with Down's syndrome have a significantly lower DBH activity compared with two control groups, one comprising non-Mongoloid mentally retarded children from the same institution ($P < 0.001$) and the other comprising normal children ($P < 0.001$). In fact, 5 of 12 children with Down's syndrome showed no detectable enzyme activity. The low plasma DBH activity does not seem to be due to the presence of an endogenous enzyme inhibitor. Plasma from children with Down's syndrome was added to plasma with normal DBH activity. This did not reduce the enzyme activity of the normal plasma. The non-Mongoloid mentally retarded children had significantly lower DBH activ-

Table 1

Dopamine-β-hydroxylase activity in the plasma of patients with Down's syndrome and of controls.

Age range	No. of cases	Diagnosis	DBH activity
3, 14 days	2	Down's syndrome	0 and 1
0 days	15	Healthy newborns	3 ± 1
5–15 years	10	Down's syndrome	4 ± 2
5–15 years	10	Non-Mongoloid mentally retarded children	46 ± 12
5–15 years	14	Normal controls	103 ± 12
20–43 years	10	Down's syndrome	67 ± 17
20–39 years	52	Normal controls	98 ± 9

The activity of DBH is mean ± SEM and is expressed in nanomoles of octopamine formed from tyramine per ml plasma per 20 min incubation time.

ity in plasma than did normal controls ($P < 0.01$).

The plasma activity of DBH in adult patients with Down's syndrome did not differ significantly from the activity found in a control group of apparently healthy individuals ($0.2 > P > 0.1$). The newborn patients with Down's syndrome as well as healthy newborns (cord blood plasma) had very low or no measurable DBH activity. The DBH activity in plasma may, at least in part, emanate from sympathetic nerves and the adrenal medulla from which it is released together with noradrenaline (Weinshilboum & Axelrod 1971 b, Weinshilboum et al. 1971). The consistently low plasma DBH activity in children with Down's syndrome could be a result of reduced activity in the sympathetic nervous system, which might indicate a fundamental dysfunction of catecholamine metabolism in this disease.

A recent report from Axelrod's laboratory showed that the plasma activity in a normal population increased with age and reached adult levels during the decade 10 to 19 years of age (Weinshilboum & Axelrod 1971 c). The findings that children with Down's syndrome aged 5 to 15 had as low a plasma DBH activity as newborns, and that adults with Down's syndrome had near normal plasma DBH, indicate that the maturation of the sympathetic nervous system may be slower in patients with this disease.

There are indications of delayed maturation in other organ systems in the children with Down's syndrome, e.g. the development of the skeleton, which coincides temporally with the slow increase in plasma DBH activity with increasing age (Hall 1965).

The possible disturbance in the synthesis or release of noradrenaline as reflected by the very low plasma DBH activity in children with Down's syndrome and the decreased DBH activity in non-Mongoloid mentally retarded children, calls for further studies of the catecholamine metabolism in children with mental retardation in general and especially in children with Down's syndrome. The results of such studies might possibly be of value in the treatment of children with Down's syndrome.

References

Bazelon, M., Paine, R. S., Cowie, V. A., Hunt, P., Houck, J. C. & Mahanand, D. (1967). Reversal of hypotonia in infants with Down's syndrome by administration of 5-hydroxytryptophan. *Lancet* i, 1130–1133.

Hall, B. (1965). Delayed ontogenesis in human trisomy syndromes. *Hereditas (Lund)* **52**, 334–344.

Rosner, F., Ong, B. H., Paine, R. S. & Mahanand, D. (1965). Blood-serotonin activity in trisomic and translocation Down's syndrome. *Lancet* i, 1191–1193.

Weinshilboum, R. & Axelrod, J. (1971a). Serum dopamine-β-hydroxylase activity. *Circulat. Res.* **28**, 307–315.

Weinshilboum, R. & Axelrod, J. (1971b). Serum dopamine-β-hydroxylase: decrease after chemical sympathectomy. *Science* **173**, 931–934.

Weinshilboum, R. & Axelrod, J. (1971c). Reduced plasma dopamine-β-hydroxylase activity in familial dysautonomia. *N. Engl. J. Med.* **285**, 938–942.

Weinshilboum, R., Kvetansky, R., Axelrod, J. & Kopin, I. J. (1971). Elevation of serum dopamine-β-hydroxylase activity with forced immobilization. *Nature New Biol.* **230**, 287–288.

An Analysis Procedure Illustrated on a Triple Linkage of Use for Prenatal Diagnosis of Myotonic Dystrophy

J. H. RENWICK and D. R. BOLLING

Diagnosis of a number of simple genetic conditions in man is now feasible prenatally (Nadler, 1971 and others) hence, for the first time, parents sometimes have the opportunity of requesting a selective abortion. For those simple genetic conditions that cannot be so diagnosed by direct means, indirect diagnosis through the prenatal phenotype for a marker locus known to be linked to the disease locus (Edwards, 1956; Renwick, 1969), is a useful substitute with potentially wide applicability. A special case is the use, in certain families, of the chromosomal sex of the embryo to give a 50% or 0% prognosis of haemophilia for male and female respectively. Attention is now drawn to an autosomal linkage between the myotonic dystrophy locus (*Dm*) and the ABH secretor locus (*Se*) that can be used in favourable circumstances to predict fairly accurately the outcome of a particular pregnancy in a family with this dystrophy.

A method of three-locus analysis was required in this work because an additional locus, *Lu* (for the Lutheran blood group), was involved. Much of the present report concerns an extension—very suitable for this purpose—of a standard Bayesian two-locus analysis (Renwick, 1969, based on Smith, 1959).

Data

On sib-pair analysis of linkage data on the pedigrees of Thomasen (1948), Mohr (1954) found indications of linkage of *Dm* with *Se* as scored from the Lewis red-cell phenotype. He found a similar indication with the Lutheran blood group locus (*Lu*), which, in turn, he knew to be linked to *Se* (Mohr, 1954; Cook, 1965).

A comprehensive, computer-based analysis has now clarified the real strength of the evidence and has encouraged collection of a further sample. The confirmation afforded by this is the subject of a separate report (Renwick *et al*, 1971), which also deals with certain problems of scoring the dystrophy and ABH secretion genotypes.

Genetic Model Underlying the Analysis

Some of the assumptions and approximations underlying linkage analysis in man are discussed by Renwick (1971). Only a few of these points require mention here.

(1) Intervals between loci are customarily measured as map-lengths because these are additive, whereas recombination fractions cannot be combined in a simple fashion over neighbouring intervals, unless these are short.

(2) A morgan is the map-length of any segment of a recovered chromosome strand that has experienced, on average, one crossover event in one meiosis.

(3) Chromatid interference is believed to be at a high level in man, leading to the mapping function, $4w = \tan^{-1} 2\theta + \tanh^{-1} 2\theta$, where w morgans is the map-length of an interval that gives a recombination fraction, θ.

(4) In women, the susceptibility to crossing-over is, for at least one and perhaps for most autosomal regions, higher than in men (Renwick, 1968). If consistency is provisionally assumed, the current estimate of the ratio, female:male, is 1·40 (95% probability limits 1·04 and 1·98) from unpublished calculations of J. H. Renwick and D. R. Bolling on data from many laboratories.

(5) The total autosomal map-length, T, based on chiasma counts will be taken to be $27\frac{1}{2}$ morgans in men. (This is an overestimate, hence it errs slightly on the side of safety in reducing the posterior odds on syntenic hypotheses.) The susceptibility-ratio estimate, 1·4, implies a map-length of about $38\frac{1}{2}$ morgans in women.

(6) Meiotic studies in men (M. Hultén, personal communication; P. L. Pearson, personal communication) show more chiasmata on long autosomes than on short ones. The approximation is here made that the relationship is a linear one. The physical lengths given by the Chicago Conference (1966) then offer a basis for partitioning the total autosomal map-length among the autosomal pairs of chromosomes. The resulting estimate of the map-length of the ith chromosome pair will be denoted by A_i and will be used in calculating prior probabilities as if it were the true value.

Bayesian Analysis for Three Loci

An analysis appropriate for multiple loci has been presented by Bolling (1970). Only the three-locus analysis will be given here but the same computer program embraces also the four-locus analysis. A brief outline of the Bayesian framework will be followed by a description of the procedure in more detail.

Prior Probabilities. The prior probability of three autosomal loci being on the same chromosome (3-synteny) is $\Sigma(A_i/T)^3$ or about 3/900. The prior probability of 2-on, 1-off (2-synteny; 1-asynteny) is $3\Sigma(A_i/T)^2(T-A_i)/T$ or $3\Sigma(A_i/T)^2 - 3\Sigma(A_i/T)^3$. (This happens to be three times the difference between the probabilities for 2-synteny and for 3-synteny.) Its numerical value is about 138/900. In Tables I and II this is partitioned equally between three options, in each of which a different locus is left out of the syntenic group. The probability for 3-synteny is likewise partitioned equally between the three possible orderings of the loci (ignoring orientation throughout). The remaining hypothesis (asynteny), under which all three loci are on different autosomes, carries the remaining probability, 759/900.

Contributions of the Data. The theorem of Bayes (1763) can be stated in terms of odds as follows: the odds on a hypothesis in the light of observations are proportional to the probability of those observations given the hypothesis multiplied by the prior odds on this hypothesis. In the present problem, the asyntenic hypothesis remains simple but the syntenic ones must be considered as composite comprising a multitude of sub-hypotheses. There is one of these sub-hypotheses for each pair of values of the map-lengths of adjacent intervals when a given order of the three loci is considered.

From the pedigree data, we calculate on a simple Mendelian model the relative probability of finding these data if there is a true recombination fraction θ_a between Dm and Se; θ_b between Se and Lu; θ_c between Dm and Lu. To have a constant standard for comparison, we standardize these odds (to antilods) by relating them to the probability when $\theta_a = \theta_b = \theta_c = \frac{1}{2}$—ie, when the loci are on different chromosomes, for example. We shall write the map-lengths corresponding to $\theta = \frac{1}{2}$ arbitrarily as $w = 1000M$: they are more correctly infinite—the loci are asyntenic and there is, at least notionally, an infinite amount of crossing-over between them.

We suppose that w_1 (the length of the $Dm:Se$ interval) yields the recombination fraction θ_a; w_2 (the $Se:Lu$ map-length) yields θ_b; w_3 (the $Dm:Lu$ map-length) yields θ_c. As already mentioned, the map-length and recombination fraction are taken to be related by the Carter-Falconer mapping function of the form: $4w = \tan^{-1}2\theta + \tanh^{-1}2\theta$. For asynteny, $\theta_a = \theta_b = \theta_c = \frac{1}{2}$; the antilod is then 1 by the standardization procedure.

Fortuitously, with one exception in Mohr's data (1954) to be considered later, no mating segregates fruitfully for more than two of the loci. The antilods from them are therefore largely indifferent to the lengths of the other intervals. Thus, for a given ordering $Dm:Se:Lu$, the antilod (denoted by α_{12}) for any pair of values of w_1 and w_2 (implying $w_3 = w_1 + w_2$) is given by

$$\alpha_{12}(D|w_1, w_2, w_3) = \alpha(D_1|w_1) \cdot \alpha(D_2|w_2) \cdot \alpha(D_3|w_3)$$

where D_1 D_2 and D_3 are non-overlapping parts that constitute the total data, D.

The lods (denoted by z) are obtained by taking logarithms with base 10:

$$z_{12}(D|w_1, w_2, w_3) = z(D_1|w_1) + z(D_2|w_2) + z(D_3|w_3).$$

Non-independence. The exceptional mating is in Pedigree 4 of Mohr's data. The children of I.34 can be scored for recombination between Dm and Se; Se and Lu; Lu and Dm simultaneously, as she is probably heterozygous. The data, D', cannot here be split into three non-overlapping parts, each relevant to a single interval. Fortunately, to achieve an approximate adjustment, we can use the following argument:

For a given ordering, say $Dm:Se:Lu$ (when w_1 and w_2 are the primary variables)

$$\alpha_{12}(D'|w_1, w_2, w_3) = \alpha(D'|w_1) \cdot \alpha(D'|w_2).$$

To gain a degree of symmetry and hence independence of the ordering we write this as follows:

$$\alpha_{12}(D'|w_1, w_2, w_3)$$
$$= [\alpha(D'|w_1) \cdot \alpha(D'|w_2) \cdot \alpha(D'|w_3)] \div \alpha(D'|w_3)$$

or, in logarithmic terms,

$$z_{12}(D'|w_1, w_2, w_3)$$
$$= [z(D'|w_1) + z(D'|w_2) + z(D'|w_3)] - z(D'|w_3).$$

That part of the expression that is enclosed in square brackets is symmetrical in w_1, w_2, w_3. It is therefore independent of order and is the same in z_{13} and z_{23} as in z_{12}. In this particular sibship, the remaining term also happens to have approximately the same numerical value whether it is $z(D'|w_3)$ for z_{12} or $z(D'|w_2)$ for z_{13} or $z(D'|w_1)$ for z_{23}. (The interdependence of the coupling phases of the three loci has been ignored but the resulting error is probably trivial in this instance.) It is convenient to rewrite each expression in terms of an adjustment, c, to each lod where $c \simeq -(1/3)z(D'|w_3) \simeq -z_1(3,0)/3$; eg, $z_{12}(D'|w_1,w_2,w_3,) = [z(D'|w_1) + c] + [z(D'|w_2) + c] + [z(D'|w_3) + c]$.

We may paraphrase this argument for events in a single meiosis as follows: For any ordering, the data concerning the two intervals that are contiguous are independent of each other; but the data on the joint interval are entirely determined by the data (from this meiosis) on the other two and must be discounted. In the raw analysis, the offspring of I.34 comprise roughly three recombinants or three non-recombinants—the lods are $z_1(3,0)$—for each of the three pairs of loci. As the three orders are taken to be equally likely, the appropriate adjustment involves the discounting of one third of these lods for each of the three pairs. This is approximately achieved by addition of the adjustment, c.

Posterior Probabilities. For each ordering of the loci, an appropriate prior density, as discussed later, can be combined with the three antilods for trial values of the true map-lengths, to yield points on a posterior unnormed probability surface. Integration over all possible values of these map-lengths gives the volume under the surface and this represents the posterior unnormed probability of the corresponding syntenic hypothesis. Estimates of map-lengths and their limits, conditional on a given sequence of loci, are readily obtained from the appropriate marginal distribution. This procedure of partitioning a hypothesis into a multitude of exhaustive and non-overlapping sub-hypotheses, each with its characteristic pair of map-length values, and then applying Bayes' argument, is essentially that introduced into the genetic field by Smith (1959).

In order to try to isolate the various components of the calculations, we calculate the 'change in the odds' or an 'averaged antilod', Λ', by dividing the posterior integral of a specified part of the distribution by the corresponding prior integral. This averaged antilod is not free of prior elements since we have, in effect, used them as weights in the averaging procedure.

Detailed Procedure

Joint Prior Probability Distribution of Interval Lengths. Let the total autosomal map length be T morgans.

Let the length of the ith autosome be $A_i > A_{i+1}$ morgans, where $0 < i < 22$.

3-synteny. Let the map-lengths FG, GH, FH, between three loci be w_1, w_2, and w_3 morgans respectively. The ordering FGH is called 12 (because the component lengths are w_1, w_2); GHF is 23; HFG is 31. From equation 4 of Irwin (1955), it follows that that part of the joint probability density for w_1, w_2, w_3, that concerns the synteny of the loci in a specific ordering on a known autosome, i, is:

$$f_i(w_1, w_2, w_3) = 2[A_i - \max(w_1, w_2, w_3)]T^{-3}$$
$$\text{if } 0 \leqslant \max(w_1, w_2, w_3) \leqslant A_i$$
$$= 0 \quad \text{if } A_i \leqslant \max(w_1, w_2, w_3) \leqslant A_1.$$

The combined limits, $0 - A_1$, demarcate the syntenic part of a distribution. (Over all values that lie within these limits and over all three orderings, this part integrates to $[A_i/T]^3$—the prior probability that three autosomal loci, chosen effectively at random, *are* on this ith autosome.)

When the loci are syntenic in the specified ordering but the autosome is *not* specified, the prior density is:

$$f(w_1, w_2, w_3) = \sum_{i=1}^{22} f_i(w_1, w_2, w_3)$$
$$0 \leqslant \max(w_1, w_2, w_3) \leqslant A_1.$$

Over all values that lie within the limits $0 - A_1$, the partial distribution described by this density function integrates, appropriately, to $\frac{1}{3}\sum_{i=1}^{22}(A_i/T)^3$, the prior probability of autosomal 3-synteny with ordering specified—about 1/900.

For each ordering, $\max(w_1, w_2, w_3)$ is always the sum of the other two lengths, hence $f(w_1, w_2, w_3)$ may be presented graphically in a bivariate form, with these two shorter lengths as the primary variables. It constitutes a surface of 22 planes of progressively decreasing tilt as shown in Fig. 1 for the ordering 12. The line of mutual intersection of any two of these is parallel to the line, $w_1 + w_2 = A_1$, in which the final plane meets the base. This diagonal line in the base is the limit beyond which the conjunct interval would exceed the length, A_1, of the longest chromosome (No. 1). As already mentioned, the proportional autosomal map-lengths (A_i/T) have been taken to be equal to the proportional physical lengths at mitotic metaphase. We now consider the only other parts of the joint

188

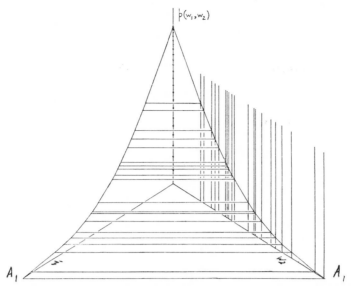

Fig. 1. The prior probability surface for the ordering $Dm:Se:Lu$ for lengths of two adjacent intervals, w_1 and w_2, on an unknown autosome. The surface consists of 22 planes of decreasing tilt intersecting each other in lines parallel to the line $w_1 + w_2 = A_1$ where A_1 is the map length of No. 1 chromosome (the longest). The surface represents only the 3-syntenic part of the distribution of map-interval lengths.

distribution of map-lengths that have non-zero prior densities. These parts involve asynteny but we may avoid the introduction of a two-valued 'tenic' variable by adopting the convention that an interval between asyntenic loci is ascribed a length of 1000 morgans except when the additivity rule of map-lengths requires it to be longer. We may partially justify this device. In a formal sense, the independent assortment of loci on different pairs of autosomes produces the same proportion of gametes that are recombinant for these loci as would be produced by an infinite amount of crossing-over between syntenic loci. The interval between chromosome pairs might indeed be regarded as one of infinite susceptibility to 'crossing-over' so that physical continuity was constantly being disrupted. Formally, then, the map-length between asyntenic loci is infinite but there are important advantages in substituting an arbitrarily large value such as 1000 morgans: addition of map-lengths is, for one thing, still meaningful.

2-synteny and its part of the distribution. There

are again three possible orderings of the loci, here depending on which one is asyntenic. This one will be written as the last locus: for example, the ordering 12 (FGH or GFH) then implies that F and G are syntenic, H is not. $\text{Min}(w_1, w_2, w_3)$ denotes the map distance between the two syntenic loci. For a specific ordering, the joint prior distribution of map-lengths has a contribution, $f_i(w_1, w_2, w_3)$, that arises when the syntenic loci are on the ith autosome:

$$f_i(w_1, w_2, w_3)$$
$$= 2[A_i - \min(w_1, w_2, w_3)]T^{-2}(T - A_i)T^{-1}$$
$$\quad \text{if } 1000 \leqslant \max(w_1, w_2, w_3) \leqslant 1000 + A_i$$
$$= 0$$
$$\quad \text{if } 1000 + A_i \leqslant \max(w_1, w_2, w_3) \leqslant 1000 + A_1.$$

(For this specific ordering and for this ith chromosome and over all values that lie within either of these sets of limits, the corresponding part of the distribution that is described by this density function integrates appropriately to $[A_i/T]^2 - [A_i/T]^3$. This is the probability that two specific loci lie on the ith autosome and that the third lies elsewhere.)

When the autosome on which the two loci are syntenic is *not* specified (the usual case), the prior density is:

$$f(w_1, w_2, w_3) = \sum_{i=1}^{22} f_i(w_1, w_2, w_3).$$

That part of the distribution for which this density is appropriate integrates to $\sum_{i=1}^{22} [(A_i/T)^2 - (A_i/T)^3]$. Its numerical value is about 46/900. The full distribution includes of course three such parts, one for each 'ordering' specifying which locus is asyntenic.

Asynteny of all three loci. The probability for asynteny is about 759/900 as already mentioned and is not distributed.

Averaged Antilod and Posterior Distribution. For a specific ordering of the loci, one interval length is completely defined by the sum of the other two, hence it does not make any non-redundant contribution to the prior densities. The data D may, however, refer to all three intervals largely in an independent and non-overlapping manner and, accordingly, may be considered in three parts—D_1, D_2, and D_3. The posterior probability density (unnormed) for interval lengths, w_1, w_2, w_3, in ordering 12 (where $w_3 = w_1 + w_2$) is therefore the algebraic product of the three likeli-

hood ratios, $\alpha(D_1|w_1)$, $\alpha(D_2|w_2)$, $\alpha(D_3|w_3)$, and the prior joint density $f_{12}(w_1, w_2, w_3)$.

The above presentation differs superficially from that of Bolling (1970) which is in terms of *conditional* distributions.

Se **Linkage Group: An Illustration of the Method.** The lods were computed for the *Dm*: *Se*, *Dm*: *Lu*, and *Se*: *Lu* intervals from all the available published and unpublished pedigree data by the program of Renwick and Schulze (1961). They are given in Table I of Renwick *et al* (1971)—for the equal-susceptibility situation, ie, when male and female map-lengths are taken to be equal.

For a specific ordering of the loci, the volume of the 3-syntenic part of the posterior probability distribution (unnormed) was determined from these three sets of total lods by the MAPIN computer program (Bolling, 1970). MAPIN is written in Fortran IV and uses two numerical integration methods which usually show good agreement with each other. The ratio of this volume to the prior volume is the averaged antilod, $\varLambda'$, or the change in the odds, for this particular ordering of the loci. The procedure was repeated for the other possible orderings.

In Table I, these values of $\varLambda'$ obtained from Mohr's data (1954) are set out for each synteny hypothesis. Those for the 2-synteny hypotheses

TABLE I

BAYESIAN ANALYSIS OF MOHR'S DATA (1954) ON LINKAGE RELATIONSHIPS OF *Dm*, *Se*, *Lu*, LOCI
(A colon separates the symbols of syntenic loci; an oblique stroke (virgule) separates the symbols of asyntenic loci.)

Hypothesis	Loci	Prior Odds	Change in Odds	Posterior Odds		Posterior Probability
3-synteny	Dm: Se: Lu	1	3.0×10^{19}	3.0×10^{19}		
	Dm: Lu: Se	1	2.2×10^{19}	2.2×10^{19}	6.8×10^{19}	0.93
	Lu: Dm: Se	1	1.6×10^{19}	1.6×10^{19}		
2-synteny	(Lu: Se)/Dm	46	1.1×10^{17}	0.5×10^{19}		
	(Dm: Se)/Lu	46	6	276 only	0.5×10^{19}	0.07
	(Dm: Lu)/Se	46	14	644 only		
asynteny	Lu/Se/Dm	759	1	759 only		
Any of these . . .		900	. . .	7.3×10^{19}	7.3×10^{19}	1.00

TABLE II

BAYESIAN ANALYSIS OF MOHR'S DATA SUPPLEMENTED BY THOSE OF RENWICK *ET AL* (1971)

Hypothesis	Loci	Prior Odds	Change in Odds	Posterior Odds		Posterior Probability
3-synteny	Dm: Se: Lu	1	30.6×10^{19}	30.6×10^{19}		
	Lu: Dm: Se	1	20.4×10^{19}	20.4×10^{19}	55.4×10^{19}	0.99
	Dm: Lu: Se	1	4.4×10^{19}	4.4×10^{19}		
2-synteny	(Lu: Se)/Dm	46	1.2×10^{17}	0.6×10^{19}		
	(Dm: Se)/Lu	46	23	1058 only	0.6×10^{19}	0.01
	(Dm: Lu)/Se	46	14	644 only		
asynteny	Lu/Se/Dm	759	1	759 only		
Any of these . . .		900	. . .	56.0×10^{19}	56.0×10^{19}	1.00

The odds on the 3-syntenic orderings, *Dm*:*Se*:*Lu*, *Lu*:*Dm*:*Se*, *Dm*:*Lu*:*Se*, are seen to be left at 30:20:4 or about 6:4:1.

were computed, for strict comparability, on the 3-synteny model with the invention of a dummy as an extra syntenic locus on which the data do not bear. (All orderings were, of course, again considered.) Mohr's data alone yielded final odds on 3-synteny of 12:1 over all other hypotheses. With the inclusion of the data of Renwick *et al* (1971), these odds became 92:1 (Table II), corresponding to a posterior probability of 0·99 that the dystrophia

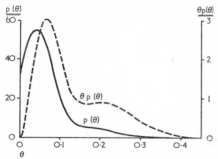

Fig. 2. Posterior distribution, $p(\theta)\,d\theta$, of the recombination fraction, θ, between *Dm* and *Se*, summed over all three orders of the loci, *Dm*, *Se*, *Lu*. The scale is unnormed. This distribution is derived from the marginal distribution of the corresponding map interval.

The graph of $\theta p(\theta)$ is also given (on a 20-fold scale shown on the right). The ratio of the areas under these two graphs, corrected for scale, is the overall probability of a recombinant,

$$P(R) = \frac{\int_0^{0·5} \theta \cdot p(\theta) \cdot d\theta}{\int_0^{0·5} p(\theta) \cdot d\theta} = 0·073.$$

locus belongs to the *Se:Lu* linkage group. Given 3-synteny, the current odds on the alternative sequences, *Dm:Se:Lu*, *Dm:Lu:Se*, *Se:Dm:Lu*, are found to be 6:4:1.

The marginal distributions were also computed by MAPIN. That for the longest interval was constructed by integrating the distribution along lines parallel to $w_1 + w_2 = A_1$ for the ordering 12; or along equivalent lines otherwise. As expected, the shape of the marginal distribution for one of the intervals—the *Lu:Se* interval—is so dominated by the data bearing directly on it that it remains almost invariant whatever the ordering of the loci, whereas the marginal distributions for the *Dm:Se* and *Dm:Lu* interval lengths reflect fewer data and therefore vary considerably among the three possible orderings.

The aggregate of the three marginal distributions for the *Dm:Se* interval gives a most probable map-length of 0·04 morgans between the two loci. The

distribution of the corresponding recombination fraction, θ (see Fig. 2) is critical when we apply these data in prenatal diagnosis as explained later.

A joint analysis (such as that outlined in this paper) is required not only to estimate each interval-length using all the data but to assess too the probability that *Dm* does indeed belong to the *Se:Lu* linkage group. This follows from the mutuality of the lengths of the three intervals, one being the sum of the other two. The powerful influences of the prior probabilities are, in themselves, good reasons for this joint analysis being of Bayesian type.

Antenatal Prediction of Myotonic Dystrophy. It was mentioned in the introduction that linkages can theoretically be used for indirect diagnosis *in utero*. The dystrophia:secretor linkage is one of the first autosomal examples. An important requirement has been met by the recent finding by Harper and Hutchinson (1970) that the amniotic fluid does reflect the secretor genotype of the fetus. (That study was stimulated by our analysis of Mohr's data.) In certain suitable families in which the affected parent is heterozygous for both loci, it should be possible to infer what allele was transmitted from the dystrophy locus from knowledge of what allele was transmitted from the secretor locus. The security of the inference would, of course, depend on the risk that the gamete was recombinant. This risk $P(R)$ would be equal to the *true* recombination fraction θ. This remains unknown but we do possess in the light of the linkage data a probability distribution for the values it might take. We cannot justifiably take the modal estimate of θ in place of its true value because the distribution is skewed markedly (towards high values of θ). Pursuing such reasoning, we take the posterior probability, $P(R)$, that a particular gamete will be recombinant for alleles at the dystrophy and secretor loci to be the sum of elements of conditional probability, $p(R|\theta)d\theta$, each weighted by the posterior probability density, $p(\theta)$, appropriate for recombination fractions lying between θ and $\theta + d\theta$. For sufficiently small increment, $d\theta$,

$$P(R) = \int_0^{0·5} p(R|\theta) \cdot p(\theta) \cdot d\theta = \int_0^{0·5} \theta p(\theta) \cdot d\theta.$$

We require, therefore, the centre of gravity (ie, the mean) of the posterior distribution of θ. We can obtain it graphically by plotting the $\theta p(\theta) \cdot d\theta$ function against θ and integrating it. To do this, we measure the area under it and the area under the distribution itself. After allowance for scaling (such as the 20-fold scaling used in Fig. 2) the ratio

191

of the areas which is found to be about 0·073 is the required probability if, on the one hand, there is synteny of Dm and Se (probability 0·99). If, on the other hand, this condition of synteny does not hold (probability 0·01), the recombination fraction is exactly 0·5. Using the combined data of the present work and of Mohr (1954), we therefore assess the probability that any specified gamete is a recombinant as $0·99(0·073) + 0·01(0·5)$ or 0·078. The probability that it is a non-recombinant is thus about 92%—so a prediction, that could be given with 100% security but for recombination, has about 92% security when we take recombination into account.

It might seem, at first sight, that the probability of a recombinant, contrary to the above, should be equal to the probability of recombination, as estimated modally from the data. If the estimate of θ were associated with only a trivial bias or only a trivial variance this would indeed be approximately true. In more real situations, all possible values of θ must be considered with weights proportional to their posterior probability densities. This can perhaps be better understood by means of an artificial oversimplification:

Consider that only three values, 0·05, 0·1, 0·2 are possible with posterior probabilities 0·7, 0·2, 0·1 respectively. The most probable recombination fraction would then be 0·05 but the probability, $P(R)$, of a particular gamete being a recombinant would be

$$P(R) = (0·7)(0·05) + (0·2)(0·1) + (0·1)(0·2) = 0·075.$$

Influence of Sex. The $Se:Lu$ region is known to be one of those that have an excess of crossing-over in females. If this region and its neighbours are average in this respect, we could perhaps use, for its female:male ratio of susceptibility to crossing-over, the overall estimate, 1·40, that we obtained recently from an unpublished analysis of available data on a number of autosomal linkages. To a first approximation, we can then derive map-length and recombination estimates for males by multiplying the above raw estimates by 5/6 and for females by multiplying by 7/6. The security of prediction is then, for a father, $100 - (7·8)(5/6)$ or 93% and, for a mother, $100 - 7·8(7/6)$ or 91%.

The main approximation involved here lies in the fact that the raw estimates are based partly on data relevant to male meiosis and partly on data relevant to female meiosis. These two sets of data can be expected in general to be unequal in size and moment, so that raw estimates obtained by pooling them are only approximations to the required un-weighted average of male and female estimates

separately derived. A more sophisticated analysis may be envisaged. It would be possible to compute these estimates subject to the current estimate of the overall susceptibility ratio if this ratio were deemed approximately uniform and therefore appropriate to this chromosomal region.

Summary

Re-analysis of data of Thomasen (1948) and Mohr (1954) that was undertaken as part of a wider computer-based linkage analysis gave evidence that the loci of myotonic dystrophy (Dm), ABH secretion (Se), and the Lutheran blood group system (Lu) might be on the same chromosome (syntenic). Like Mohr, who made the same observation by a different method, we should have found the evidence difficult to evaluate but for a fortuitous concurrence with the designing of a Bayesian computer analysis for linkage data involving 3 or 4 loci. Extension to 5 loci appears feasible but extension to 6 without further approximation does not. That method is published for the first time here.

The posterior probability, 0·93, that the 3 loci are syntenic stimulated collection of further data that now raise it to 0·99 (Renwick et al, 1971). The method when applied to these two sets of data, gives a preferred map $Dm:Se:Lu$ with consecutive intervals of lengths 0·04:0·13 morgans, though other orderings are also possible.

The $Dm:Se$ linkage is important since it can be used for an indirect and novel form of prenatal diagnosis. In suitable pedigrees, the dystrophia can be predicted with 92% security on the basis of the secretor phenotype of the fetus as determined on its amniotic fluid (Harper and Hutchinson, 1970).

Drs E. A. Murphy and Helen Abbey, and Professors M. J. M. Bernal and P. Armitage made material contributions to the development of the method. The work was carried out chiefly in London in 1969 during part of the tenure by D.R.B. of a training award from the US Public Health Service. It was supported also by grants G968/206B from the Medical Research Council and GM-10189 from the National Institutes of Health (Dr V. A. McKusick, Johns Hopkins Hospital Medical School, Baltimore). The program was developed on the CDC 6600 computer of the University of London Computing Centre through the Birkbeck terminal.

REFERENCES

Bayes, T. (1763). An essay towards solving a problem in the doctrine of chances. *Philosophical Transactions of the Royal Society*, **53**, 370–418. Reprinted in *Biometrika* (1958), **45**, 293–315.

Bolling, D. R. (1970). *The Multi-point Mapping of Gene Loci in Man.* MSc Thesis, Johns Hopkins University.

Chicago Conference: Standardization in Human Cytogenetics (1966).

Birth Defects: Original Article Series, II, 2, p. 3. National Foundation—March of Dimes, New York.

Cook, P. J. L. (1965). The Lutheran-Secretor recombination fraction in man: a possible sex difference. *Annals of Human Genetics*, 28, 393–401.

Edwards, J. H. (1956). Antenatal detection of hereditary disorders. *Lancet*, 2, 579.

Harper, P. and Hutchinson, J. R. (1970). ABO secretor status of the fetus in early pregnancy—a genetic marker identifiable by amniocentesis. (Abstr.) *American Journal of Human Genetics*, 22, 41a–42a.

Irwin, J. O. (1955). A unified derivation of some well-known frequency distributions of interest in biometry and statistics. *Journal of the Royal Statistical Society*, 118, 389–404.

Mohr, J. (1954). A study of linkage in man. (*Opera ex Domo Biologiae Hereditariae Humanae Universitatis Hafniensis*, vol. 33.) Munksgaard, Copenhagen.

Nadler, H. L. (1971). Indications for amniocentesis in the early prenatal detection of genetic disorders. *Birth Defects: Original Article Series*, VII, 5, p. 5. National Foundation — March of Dimes, New York.

Renwick, J. H. (1968). Ratios of female to male recombination fractions in man. *Bulletin of the European Society of Human Genetics*, 2, 7–14.

Renwick, J. H. (1969). Widening the scope of antenatal diagnosis. *Lancet*, 2, 386.

Renwick, J. H. (1971). The mapping of human chromosomes. *Annual Review of Genetics*, 5. (In press.)

Renwick, J. H., Bundey, S. E., Ferguson-Smith, M.A., and Izatt, M.M. (1971). Confirmation of linkage of the loci for myotonic dystrophy and ABH secretion. *Journal of Medical Genetics*, 8, 407–416.

Renwick, J. H. and Schulze, J. (1961). A computer programme for the processing of linkage data from large pedigrees. (Abstr.) *Excerpta Medica, International Congress Series*, 32, E145.

Smith, C. A. B. (1959). Some comments on the statistical methods used in linkage investigations. *American Journal of Human Genetics*, 11, 289–304.

Thomasen, E. (1948). Myotonia. Thomasen's disease. Paramyotonia. Dystrophia myotonica. (*Opera ex Domo Biologia Hereditariae Universitatis Humanae Hafniensis*, vol. 17.) Munksgaard, Copenhagen.

Confirmation of Linkage of the Loci for Myotonic Dystrophy and ABH Secretion

J. H. RENWICK, SARAH E. BUNDEY, M. A. FERGUSON-SMITH, and MARIAN M. IZATT

Mohr (1954) found hints that the locus of myotonic dystrophy belongs to the Secretor:Lutheran ($Se:Lu$) linkage group established by Mohr (1951). Despite their potential relevance for genetic counselling, these hints did not lead to further studies for reasons which may have revolved around the difficulties in phenotypic and genotypic categorization for the secretor and dystrophy loci. There may also have been some caution from an awareness of some limitations of the statistical procedures available at that time.

A reappraisal of the dystrophy linkage data by Renwick and Bolling (1971) arose from a routine Bayesian analysis of Mohr's data undertaken in 1968 as part of their comprehensive analysis of available linkage data. Using computer help, they assessed the linkage relationships between the three loci jointly and obtained the posterior probability that all were syntenic (on the same chromosome). This probability was 0·93.

Plans were made to collect further data and were stimulated by two further developments. One was the revival of interest (Renwick, 1969) in the indirect technique of prenatal diagnosis using a linkage relationship (Edwards, 1956). The other was the improvement in methods for early recognition of heterozygotes for the dystrophy allele. A linkage study is here reported in which a re-investigation of many of the pedigrees that had been studied for that purpose by Bundey, Carter, and Soothill (1970) increases the probability that the three loci, Dm, Se, Lu, are on the same chromosome pair (syntenic). A preliminary report has already appeared (Renwick et al, 1971).

Myotonic Dystrophy and the Pedigrees Studied

These authors studied 34 pedigrees of myotonic dystrophy with the aim of detecting, by special investigations, heterozygotes for the dystrophy allele before the age of clinical symptoms. (This age varies widely. Anamnestically and without diagnostic aid from clinical signs, it exceeds 35 years in about one third of the propositi of Lynas [1957] and also of Klein [1958].) Special tests performed on about half the clinically normal first-degree relatives showed that slit-lamp examination of the lens (through detection of characteristic multicoloured cortical opacities) and electromyography (through detection of electrical myotonia) could be used to identify heterozygotes before other clinical signs. It was considered that slit-lamp abnormalities were the earliest sign and could precede clinical manifestation by at least 6 years (Klein, 1958) and perhaps longer. The electromyogram could however be normal in the presence of lenticular opacities. A follow-up would be necessary to determine how far negative investigations in a clinically normal first-degree relative would increase the probability that he or she was not a heterozygote.

Seventeen of the 34 pedigrees were chosen for linkage studies. Some of the pedigrees have been extended.* Charts of the pedigrees studied for linkage are given on pp. 411–414. The last two digits of the pedigree code names correspond to the family numbering of the 1970 study (Bundey et al, 1970), except for DM189 which corresponds to family 31. Clinical status and results of special investigations are reported in Bundey et al (1970).

Two additional families, DM135 and DM136, were not seen in the earlier study. In DM135 the proposita III.1 had been referred for genetic counselling; in DM136 the proposita IV.6 and her affected cousin IV.3 were seen at the Hospital for Sick Children.

---

* The detailed pedigrees of certain members of the families studied, in particular those who have been tested for blood group and other polymorphic markers, can be found in the Biological Data Collection of the General Library of the British Museum (Natural History), Cromwell Road, London SW7.

DM189 had been investigated by M. d'A. Crawfurd, W. D. Fletcher, T. E. Cleghorn, E. B. Robson, and H. Harris (personal communication). A linkage study (including blood and secretor typing) had been carried out and some clinically normal relatives had undergone electromyography. Only a little further information on relatives was obtained in the present study.

The families were visited, the clinical status of each relative was verified, and blood and saliva samples were collected. A few relatives, not previously investigated, were examined by electromyography and for lenticular opacities with the Haag-Streit slit-lamp. The reason for these extra investigations was either a suspected change in clinical status or a query of a genetic counselling nature. Individuals scored as heterozygotes are those who, whatever their age, show clinical evidence of myotonic dystrophy or, who, while clinically normal, show unequivocal evidence of being heterozygous on slit-lamp or electromyographic examination. It was not possible to be certain about 'normal' individuals in view of the variation in the age of onset of signs. For the purposes of the linkage calculations, an individual has been scored as homozygous normal only if he or she shows no evidence of the dystrophy and has reached the age of 35. There are 26 such individuals in the study and 13 have, additionally, undergone slit-lamp examination and/or electromyography with no findings indicating heterozygosity for the *Dm* allele.

All individuals who are under 35 years and have an affected or potentially affected parent have been excluded from the analysis unless they are clearly heterozygotes. When some or all are old enough to be scored for their *Dm* genotypes with greater reliability, their inclusion should improve the precision of the linkage estimates.

Genetical Classification based on Clinical, Lenticular, and Myographic Findings

Bundey et al (1970) have reported the clinical findings. Subsequently, in DM1B3, III.6 has developed clinical myotonia, which was not present at the original examination 2 years previously when he was 8 years of age. He also has characteristic lenticular opacities on slit-lamp examination. His brother, III.5, without clinical myotonia, has similar lenticular opacities; neither had previously been examined with the slit-lamp. In DM189, II.14 now aged 67, who had a normal electromyogram in 1964, now has typical lenticular opacities, but no clinical myotonia. In DM134, III.4 is

clinically normal, has a normal electromyogram, but has characteristic lenticular opacities; she had not been seen previously. In DM189, I.3 aged 89 has senile cataracts, but no lenticular changes of the relevant type. In DM136, III.1 has a normal electromyogram.

There is no method for assessing accurately the extent of misclassification, particularly as the true segregation ratio may not be exactly 50:50 and as the mode of ascertainment is complex. However, it is considered that most if not all heterozygotes over 35 have been recognized. In the 19 families, among non-propositi with one affected parent, there were 111 aged 35 or over at the time of the study or at the time of death, and of these 56 were classed as affected, ie, 51%. If the examination criteria for inclusion in this series had been as restrictive as those used in the classification for linkage purposes, the proportion affected would have been, if anything, greater than this. (This confidence in the classification of heterozygotes over 35 years is enhanced by consideration of the corresponding segregation ratio in those 18 pedigrees of the first study that were not included in the second: 10 affected persons out of 20.)

Polymorphic Marker Loci

A wide range of polymorphic loci controlling erythrocyte antigens, serum proteins, cell enzymes are being tested.* Most of the methods used are based on those of Race and Sanger (1968) and on Giblett's modifications (1969) of techniques from London and elsewhere.

The Secretor Locus and its alleles *Se* and *se*.
On an erythrocyte or other human cell, the A, B, or H antigen is present as a glycosphingolipid. In genotypes having at least one *Se* allele, some of the same antigenic specificity is also built up by the ABH enzyme system as a glycoprotein. This is water-soluble and secreted in saliva and other body fluids including the amniotic fluid. Another substrate of the ABH enzyme system, in the presence of an *Se* allele, is Le^a antigen which is converted to Le^b. The Le(a−) phenotype thus indicates presence of at least one *Se* allele unless there is some block in the synthesis of Le^a substance itself. Such a block occurs in homozygotes for the *l* allele at the true Lewis locus. In most European populations the frequency of such homozygotes is about 4%. Even of these, only about 23% of the genotypes will be

---

* The results to date are available from the Biological Data Collection of the General Library of the British Museum (Natural History).

misclassified as containing at least one *Se* allele because, in the remaining 77%, the genotype will be correctly deduced to be a secreting one. Thus in a sample such as that of Mohr (1954) only 1% error (23% of 4%) is expected when the genotype is scored from the Le(a) phenotype. The elucidation of these interactions is largely the work of Grubb (1951), Ceppellini (1955), Kabat (1956), Morgan and Watkins (1969), and Watkins (1971).

The secretor locus has been satisfactorily scored on the saliva in the present study and the detectability of Le^a on erythrocytes was to be used only to confirm the absence of the *Se* allele. However owing to the poor quality of the only anti-Le^a sera available except those for DM189, the confirmatory Le(a) typing of the erythrocytes was not sufficiently reliable and is not recorded.

Mohr's Data on Myotonic Dystrophy. The pedigrees of Thomasen (1948) were tested for various blood group markers by Mohr (1954). The results from testing Lewis will be described in terms of the *Se* locus in the light of the present-day interpretations of their interactions.

Mohr detected indications of linkage of the dystrophy locus with the *Se* locus and with the *Lu* locus but, as noted above, these were not followed up. The standard error of the sib-pair linkage statistic had just been shown by Smith (1953) to be underestimated. The relationship between Lewis and Secretor had not been clarified. Another factor contributing to the lack of conviction or follow-up was the difficulty in genotyping those phenotypically unaffected by the disease. This difficulty arises from the variation in the age of onset.

A recent re-analysis of these dystrophy data by Renwick and Bolling (1970 and 1971), that involves the three loci simultaneously, yields a posterior probability of 0·93 that they are syntenic. The diagnoses made by Thomasen (1948), sometimes with assistance from slit-lamp microscopy, were used

without modification whatever the person's age. A re-examination of those persons classed as normal, followed by a repeat of the analysis, may well improve the dependability of the linkage estimates, particularly as some of those persons were under 35 years at the time of examination.

Linkage Analysis

The analysis follows that given by Renwick and Bolling (1971) for Mohr's data but the complication of non-independence of the linkage observations on the three intervals such as that allowed for in DM1.4 of those data did not arise in the present data. For convenience, the lods calculated with computer aid on Mohr's data (and the adjustment required for the non-independence mentioned above) are given here, pedigree by pedigree, together with those of the present series. The lods are given for a range of values of θ, where θ represents both the male and female recombination fractions. The implications of a sex difference in θ are discussed by Renwick and Bolling (1971).

In Table I, the lods relate to the established *Lu*:*Se* linkage (Mohr, 1951). They are based partly on our own data but mainly on pedigree data that have been kindly made available from a large number of laboratories notably those of Drs Mohr, Race, Greenwalt, Cleghorn, Harris, Lawler, and Lamm. For reasons of comparability, these lods were used for both analyses—that of Mohr's data alone and that of the combined data.

In Table II, the lods relate to the *Dm*:*Se* interval. It may be noted that in neither series is there clear evidence of even a single recombination in this interval.

In Table III, the lods relate to the *Dm*:*Lu* interval. The present series adds practically nothing here, but even on simple inspection of the lods from Mohr's data, an ordering of the loci that makes this the longest interval of the three is seen to be favoured.

TABLE I

AGGREGATE LODS FROM NUMEROUS PEDIGREES, PUBLISHED AND UNPUBLISHED, FOR *Se*:*Lu* INTERVAL

	Recombination Fraction (θ)									
	0·5	0·45	0·40	0·35	0·30	0·25	0·20	0·15	0·10	0·05	0
Lods (*Se*:*Lu*)	0	1·107	3·765	7·219	10·858	14·234	16·8C6	18·428	17·938	12·736	$-\infty$
Adjustment (*c*)	0	−0·004	−0·016	−0·035	−0·057	−0·081	−0·106	−0·131	−0·155	−0·178	−0·201
Adjusted lods	0	1·103	3·749	7·184	10·810	14·153	16·700	18·297	17·783	12·558	$-\infty$

The lods include data from the laboratories of Drs Mohr, Race, Greenwalt, Cleghorn, Harris, Lawler, Renwick, and several others. They are given for a range of values of the recombination fraction, θ, without regard to the known difference between the male and female values. The adjustment, *c*, which is occasioned by the non-independence in DM1.4 of the data on the three intervals is also shown (see text).

TABLE II

LODS FROM PEDIGREES OF MOHR (1954) AND PEDIGREES OF PRESENT SERIES FOR Dm:Se INTERVAL

Pedigree Mohr (1954)	Code Name*	Recombination Fraction (θ)						
		0·5	0·4	0·3	0·2	0·1	0·05	0
3	DM1·3	0	−0·006	−0·025	−0·059	−0·111	−0·146	−0·188
4	DM1·4	0	−0·038	0·152	0·312	0·492	0·584	0·675
	Adjustment (c)	0	−0·016	−0·057	−0·106	−0·155	−0·178	−0·201
6	DM1·6	0	0·044	0·146	0·252	0·282	0·195	−0·240
9	DM1·9	0	0·024	0·090	0·181	0·277	0·324	0·371
13	DM113	0	−0·016	−0·067	−0·153	−0·280	−0·358	−0·444
16	DM116M	0	0·147	0·428	0·702	0·943	1·052	1·153
7 11 12 14 15 18 19		0	0·003	0·012	0·022	0·023	0·017	0·005
Total lods (Mohr's study)		0	0·218	0·679	1·151	1·471	1·490	1·131
Present Study	DM1B1	0	0·026	0·096	0·192	0·299	0·353	0·407
	DM1B2	0	0·006	0·024	0·052	0·088	0·109	0·131
	DM1B3	0	0·006	0·026	0·056	0·096	0·119	0·143
	DM1B7	0	0·012	0·031	0·063	0·112	0·144	0·181
	DM1B9	0	0·025	0·096	0·199	0·320	0·384	0·448
	DM110	0	0·014	0·064	0·153	0·273	0·341	0·414
	DM127	0	−0·015	−0·017	0·025	0·109	0·156	0·200
	DM132	0	−0·014	−0·058	−0·144	−0·312	−0·465	−0·760
	DM134	0	−0·022	−0·047	−0·079	−0·120	−0·146	−0·177
	DM189	0	−0·012	−0·040	−0·077	−0·113	−0·124	−0·125
8 16 20 21 22 36		0	0·002	0·006	0·012	0·009	0·008	0·008
Total lods (present study)		0	0·028	0·181	0·452	0·761	0·879	0·870
Lods (grand total)		0	0·246	0·860	1·603	2·232	2·369	2·001

The lods are given for a range of values of the recombination fraction, θ. The adjustment, c, of the lods for DM1·4 is to allow for the non-independence of the data on the three intervals. In DM132, II.6 is not yet included in the calculation. DM135 is uninformative.
* All the pedigrees in the second half of the Table are those of the present paper.

TABLE III

LODS FROM MOHR'S PEDIGREES (1954) AND PEDIGREES OF PRESENT SERIES FOR Dm:Lu INTERVAL

Pedigree Mohr (1954)	Code Name	Recombination Fraction (θ)						
		0·5	0·4	0·3	0·2	0·1	0·05	0
4	DM1·4	0	0·255	0·612	0·894	0·946	0·747	−∞
	Adjustment (c)	0	−0·016	−0·057	−0·106	−0·155	−0·178	−0·201
12	DM112	0	−0·009	−0·035	−0·084	−0·162	−0·218	−0·289
15	DM115	0	0·457	0·800	1·030	1·086	0·949	−∞
19	DM119	0	0·009	0·033	0·071	0·120	0·146	0·174
3 6 7 11 13 14 18		0	−0·001	−0·002	−0·004	−0·006	−0·006	−0·007
Total lods (Mohr's study)		0	0·695	1·351	1·801	1·829	1·440	−∞
Total lods (present study)*		0	0·001	0·002	0·005	0·009	0·012	0·015
Lods (grand total)		0	0·696	1·353	1·806	1·838	1·452	−∞

The lods are given for a range of values of the recombination fraction, θ. The present series contributes only negligibly to these lods. The adjustment, c, of the lods for DM1·4 is to allow for the non-independence of the data on the three intervals.
* See Table II for pedigree names.

This is confirmed by the analysis summary presented in Table III which incorporates all available data from the two series. The odds on synteny of all three loci are seen to be 92:1 (ie, the probability is 0.99).

The three-locus computer analysis also gives us three distributions (for example of the Dm:Se map-length). Each is conditional on a particular ordering but since the distributions are unnormed, we have been able to combine them simply by addition to obtain an overall distribution. This has a peak in the region of 0·04M ($\theta = 0·04$). From the graph, we have found the narrowest 95% probability zone by trial and error usage of a planimeter:

197

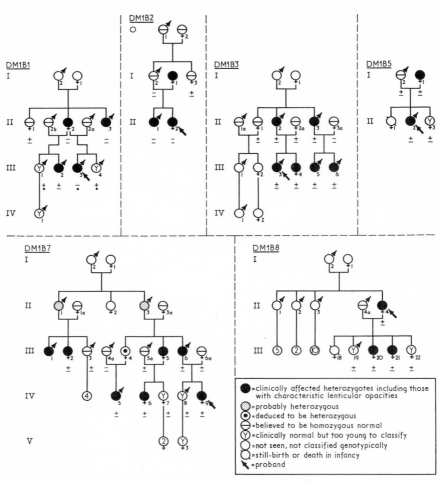

Charts of the pedigrees studied for linkage are given in this and the following three pages. The secretor phenotype (+ or −) is indicated under the number or the symbol of each tested individual and the Lu(a) phenotype is indicated below this. A dot indicates not tested.

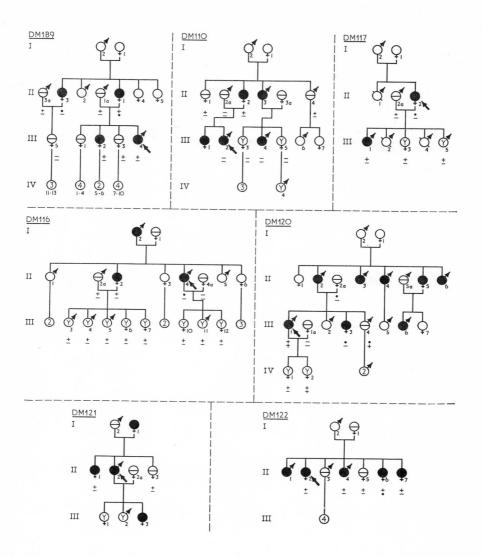

199

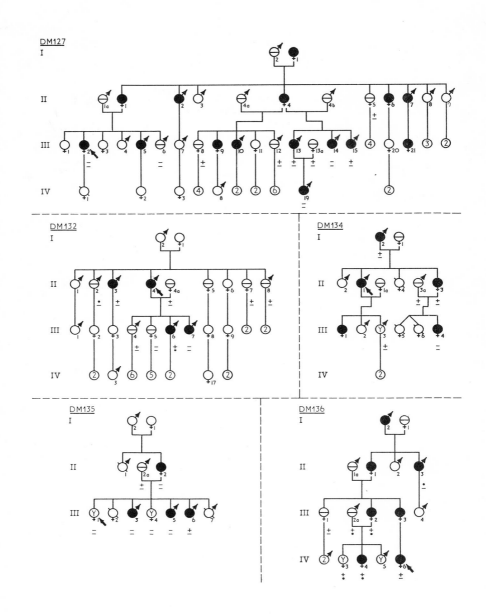

200

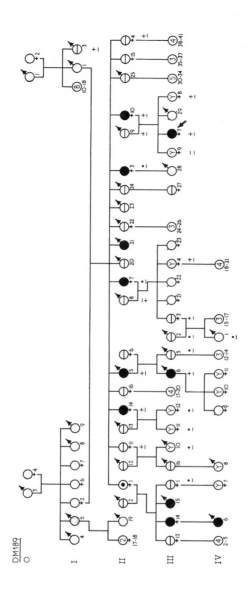

DM189

201

it extends from 0 to 0·21 morgans and corresponds to the region $0 \leqslant \theta \leqslant 0·21$.

For counselling purposes we may require the probability that a particular child is a recombinant. Renwick and Bolling (1971) explain why this probability turns out to be higher than the maximum probability estimate of θ. It is about 0·073—almost $2\hat{\theta}$ in this instance.

Clinical Significance

This is the first inherited disorder with onset in adult life, where linkage to autosomal marker loci has been found. One clinical application of such linkage will be in genetic counselling. The most valuable information can be offered in a family where the affected parent is a secretor, married to a non-secretor, and the coupling phase is known as a result of studies on other relatives. If, in this affected parent, the Dm allele is on the same homologue as the Se allele, and the clinically normal offspring is secretor negative, there would be a 100%-confident prediction of normality for that offspring, but for the possibility of genetic recombination. As explained by Renwick and Bolling (1971) the prediction still has a 92% probability of being correct even when allowance is made for recombination. If on the other hand, the offspring in such a family is secretor positive, then there is a good chance that he or she has inherited the Dm allele along with the Se allele. If, in the future, the homozygous secretor state can be distinguished from the heterozygous state, then linkage information will be helpful in a larger proportion of families.

The secretor status of the embryo may be recognized even at 9 weeks' gestation, by detection of antigens in the amniotic fluid (Harper and Hutchinson, 1970) so there may be occasions when, using similar arguments, we may assess the probability that the fetus of an affected individual has the Dm allele. In a small proportion of affected × normal matings, prenatal testing of embryonic secretor status may be useful. The parents then have the option of choosing abortion if the risk of transmission is high, in the knowledge that in a subsequent pregnancy similar tests could indicate a much smaller risk. No limitations of family size need, therefore, be involved. There are no suitable pregnancies at present in the families of the present study.

Summary

Close linkage of the autosomal loci, Dm, Se, Lu (for myotonic dystrophy, ABH secretion, and the Lutheran blood group respectively), which was adumbrated by Mohr (1954), has been established. Criteria for classification of the Dm and Se phenotypes in the study of a score of informative pedigrees are discussed with emphasis on slit-lamp microscopy and electromyography. Some important implications of the Dm:Se linkage for genetic counselling, particularly prenatally, are set out.

We are grateful to the consultants of the National Hospital for Nervous Diseases and the Hospital for Sick Children for permission to study the families of patients under their care. We thank Dr A. D. Stoker and Dr D. Smith for help with visiting members of DM135 and DM120 respectively.

The computing work was made possible by a grant from the John A. Hartford Foundation, by grant GM-10189 from the US National Institutes of Health to Dr V. A. McKusick, and by the services and facilities of the Homewood and Medical Computing Centers of Johns Hopkins University and its Medical Institutions. These are partly supported by educational contributions from the International Business Machines Corporation, and by a grant FR-00004 from the US National Institutes of Health. The data processing was supported in part by grants G960/109B and G968/206B and some of the laboratory work by G969/52B from the Medical Research Council (UK). Much of the laboratory work was supported by a grant from the Scottish Hospital Endowment Research Trust to Dr M. A. Ferguson-Smith. The technical assistance of Mrs J. Black, Mrs F. MacColl, Miss J. van den Branden, Miss S. Richards, and Miss L. Barron with particular polymorphic systems is appreciated. Mrs L. Maudling and Miss T. M. Wancowicz assisted in the data processing.

We are grateful to Dr C. O. Carter for his advice and comments during this study.

REFERENCES

Bundey, S., Carter, C. O., and Soothill, J. F. (1970). Early recognition of heterozygotes for the gene for dystrophia myotonica. *Journal of Neurology, Neurosurgery and Psychiatry*, **33**, 279–293.

Ceppellini, R. (1955). On the genetics of secretor and Lewis characters: a family study. In *Proceedings of the 5th Congress of the International Society of Blood Transfusion, Paris*, pp. 207–211.

Edwards, J. H. (1956). Antenatal detection of hereditary disorders. *Lancet*, **1**, 579.

Giblett, E. R. (1969). *Genetic Markers in Human Blood*. Blackwell, Oxford.

Grubb, R. (1951). Observations on the human blood group system Lewis. *Acta Pathologica et Microbiologica Scandinavica*, **28**, 61–81.

Harper, P. and Hutchinson, J. R. (1970). ABO secretor status of the fetus in early pregnancy—a genetic marker identifiable by amniocentesis. (Abstr.) *American Journal of Human Genetics*, **22**, 41a–42a.

Kabat, E. A. (1956). *Blood Group Substances: Their Chemistry and Immunochemistry*. Academic Press, New York.

Klein, D. (1958). La dystrophie myotonique (Steinert) et la myotonie congénitale (Thomsen) en Suisse. *Journal de Génétique Humaine*, Suppl., **7**, 1–328.

Lynas, M. A. (1957). Dystrophia myotonica with special reference to Northern Ireland. *Annals of Human Genetics*, **21**, 318–351.

Mohr, J. (1951). Estimation of linkage between the Lutheran and the Lewis blood groups. *Acta Pathologica et Microbiologica Scandinavica*, **29**, 339–344.

Mohr, J. (1954). A study of linkage in man. *Opera ex Domo Biologiae Hereditariae Humanae Universitatis Hafniensis*, Vol. 33. Munksgaard, Copenhagen.

Morgan, W. T. J. and Watkins, W. M. (1969). Genetic and bio-chemical aspects of human blood group A−, B−, H−, Le^a−, Le^b− specificity. *British Medical Bulletin*, **25**, 30–34.

Race, R. R. and Sanger, R. (1968). *Blood Groups in Man*, 5th ed. Blackwell, Oxford.

Renwick, J. H. (1969). Widening the scope of antenatal diagnosis. *Lancet*, **2**, 386.

Renwick, J. H. and Bolling, D. R. (1970). The linkage method of assignment of loci to individual autosomes. (Abstr.). *Heredity*, **25**, 150.

Renwick, J. H. and Bolling, D. R. (1971). An analysis procedure illustrated on a triple linkage of use for prenatal diagnosis of myotonic dystrophy. *Journal of Medical Genetics*, **8**, 399–406.

Renwick, J. H., Bundey, S. E., Ferguson-Smith, M. A., and Izatt, M. M. (1971). Mohr's linkage hat-trick confirmed: enables pre-natal diagnosis of myotonic dystrophy from secretor phenotype of fetus. (Abstr.) *Excerpta Medica, International Congress Series*, **233**, 150.

Smith, C. A. B. (1953). The detection of linkage in human genetics. *Journal of the Royal Statistical Society*, **2**, 153–192. Series B.

Thomasen, E. (1948). Myotonia. Thomasen's disease. Para-myotonia. Dystrophia myotonica. *Opera ex Domo Biologiae Hereditariae Humanae Universitatis Hafniensis*, Vol. 17. Munks-gaard, Copenhagen.

Watkins, W. M. (1971). In *Glycoproteins*, 2nd ed., ed. A. Gotts-chalk, Chapter 10. Elsevier, Amsterdam.

AUTHOR INDEX

KEY-WORD TITLE INDEX